Essential Oils Unveiled:

A Comprehensive Guide to Natural Healing and Wellness

Written by: Sarah Burkhartt

Essential Oils Unveiled: A Comprehensive Guide to Natural Healing and Wellness

Three Isles Publishing

www.threeislespublishing.com

Cover design by Dee Williamson

Printed in the United States of America

Disclaimer

The information provided in this book is for educational and informational purposes only. While every effort has been made to ensure the accuracy and completeness of the content, the author/publisher makes no representations or warranties of any kind, express or implied, about the completeness, accuracy, reliability, suitability, or availability of the information contained herein.

The techniques, strategies, and suggestions presented in this book are based on the author's personal experiences and research. They may not be suitable for every individual or situation. Readers are advised to use their own discretion and judgment when applying any information from this book to their own circumstances.

The author/publisher shall not be held liable for any loss, injury, or damage arising from the use of the information contained in this book. Readers are solely responsible for their own actions and decisions.

Any references to specific products, services, or organizations are provided for informational purposes only and do not constitute an endorsement or recommendation. The author/publisher shall not be held liable for any consequences resulting from the use or misuse of such products, services, or organizations.

It is recommended that readers consult with qualified professionals or experts in the relevant field before making any significant decisions or taking any actions based on the information provided in this book.

By reading this book, the reader acknowledges and agrees to the terms of this disclaimer.

Dedication

To the bold readers who've ever accidentally over-oiled a diffuser, creating a lavender fog worthy of a sci-fi movie, and to those who bravely put "just a few drops" of peppermint oil in their bath only to emerge feeling like a human candy cane—this book is for you.

May this guide help you avoid turning your home into an overwhelming botanical cloud and instead, unveil the true art and science of essential oils. Here's to discovering the perfect balance between aromatherapy bliss and olfactory overkill. Dive in, experiment wisely, and may your journey to natural healing and wellness be filled with fragrant delight and just the right amount of eucalyptus. Enjoy the ride!

Table of Content

Introduction

- *History and Evolution*

- *The Science Behind Essential Oils*

- *Benefits and Applications*

- *Purpose and Structure of the Book*

History and Evolution

The use of essential oils dates back thousands of years. Ancient civilizations such as the Egyptians, Greeks, and Romans revered these oils for their medicinal, spiritual, and cosmetic uses. The Egyptians, for instance, used essential oils in their embalming practices and for treating various ailments. They believed that these oils had the power to purify the body and mind, ensuring a smooth journey to the afterlife.

In ancient Greece, Hippocrates, the father of modern medicine, documented the therapeutic uses of aromatic oils. The Greeks utilized essential oils in their baths, massages, and medical treatments. Similarly, the Romans incorporated these precious oils into their daily lives, using them in public baths and as perfumes and medicinal remedies.

Humans' knowledge of essential oils continued to evolve during the Middle Ages, despite the decline in their use due to the fall of the Roman Empire. The Crusaders reintroduced essential oils to Europe, where they were used extensively during the Renaissance for their healing properties. The advent of modern science in the 19th century allowed for a deeper understanding of the chemical composition and therapeutic potential of essential oils, leading to the development of aromatherapy as a distinct field.

The Science Behind Essential Oils

Understanding the science behind essential oils is key to unlocking their full potential. These oils are composed of various chemical constituents such as terpenes, esters, aldehydes, ketones, and phenols, each contributing to their unique therapeutic properties. For example, linalool, found in lavender, is known for its calming effects, while limonene, found in citrus oils, is recognized for its uplifting and immune-boosting properties.

Essential oils interact with the body in several ways. When inhaled, their aromatic molecules are absorbed through the olfactory system and directly influence the brain's limbic system, which governs emotions, memory, and mood. This is why certain scents can evoke powerful emotional responses and memories.

Topical application of essential oils allows them to be absorbed through the skin and enter the bloodstream, providing localized benefits as well as systemic effects. For instance, applying peppermint oil to the temples can alleviate headaches, while eucalyptus oil can be rubbed on the chest to ease respiratory issues.

Moreover, essential oils possess antimicrobial, anti-inflammatory, and antioxidant properties, making them effective in combating infections, reducing inflammation, and protecting against oxidative stress. These scientific insights validate the centuries-old wisdom of using essential oils for health and wellness.

Benefits and Applications

The benefits of essential oils are vast and varied – as you just read – extending to nearly every aspect of health and wellness. They can be used to alleviate physical ailments, enhance emotional well-being, and even improve the environment around you. Here are some of the primary benefits and applications of essential oils:

- **Physical Health**: Essential oils can address a wide range of physical health issues. For example, tea tree oil is renowned for its antimicrobial properties, making it effective against skin infections and acne. Lavender oil is celebrated for its ability to promote relaxation and improve sleep quality. Peppermint oil can relieve digestive issues and headaches, while eucalyptus oil supports respiratory health.

- **Emotional Well-Being**: The impact of essential oils on emotional health is profound. Aromatherapy, the practice of using essential oils for therapeutic purposes, can reduce stress, anxiety, and depression. Scents like lavender, chamomile, and rose have calming effects that can soothe the mind and promote a sense of peace. Conversely, citrus oils like lemon, orange, and bergamot are uplifting and can boost mood and energy levels.

- **Environmental Enhancement**: Essential oils can also be used to purify and enhance your living spaces. Diffusing essential oils such as lemon, tea tree, and eucalyptus can cleanse the air of pathogens and provide a refreshing atmosphere. Additionally, essential oils can be incorporated into cleaning products to create a healthier, toxin-free home environment.

- **Personal Care**: Many people incorporate essential oils into their personal care routines. They can be added to skincare products to improve complexion, used in hair care to promote healthy growth, and even included in homemade bath salts and scrubs for a luxurious spa experience.

Purpose and Structure of the Book

"Essential Oils Unveiled: A Comprehensive Guide to Natural Healing and Wellness" is designed to be your go-to resource for everything related to essential oils. Whether you are a beginner just starting your journey or an experienced user looking to deepen your knowledge, this book offers valuable insights and practical advice.

The book is organized into ten comprehensive chapters, each focusing on a different aspect of essential oils:

1. **Introduction to Essential Oils**: This chapter provides a foundational understanding of what essential oils are, their history, and their basic uses.

2. **The Extraction and Production of Essential Oils**: Here, we delve into the various methods of extracting essential oils and the importance of purity and quality.

3. **Essential Oil Profiles: Popular Oils and Their Properties**: This chapter profiles some of the most popular essential oils, detailing their unique properties and benefits.

4. **Aromatherapy: The Art of Using Essential Oils**: Learn about the techniques and benefits of aromatherapy and how to create your own blends.

5. **Essential Oils for Physical Health**: Discover how essential oils can be used to address common physical health issues.

6. **Essential Oils for Mental and Emotional Well-Being**: Explore the powerful impact of essential oils on emotional health and well-being.

7. **Integrating Essential Oils into Daily Life**: Practical tips on incorporating essential oils into your personal care, home, and daily routines.

8. **Essential Oils for Specific Populations**: Guidance on using essential oils safely and effectively for children, the elderly, pregnant women, and more.

9. **Advanced Applications and Blending Techniques**: Advanced techniques for creating therapeutic blends and products.

10. **Building Your Essential Oil Toolkit**: Recommendations for essential oils, tools, and resources to build your collection and continue learning.

Additionally, the conclusion of the book reflects on your journey with essential oils, discusses the future of essential oil use, and provides resources for continued learning.

Throughout the book, you will find practical tips, DIY recipes, safety guidelines, and expert insights to help you make the most of essential oils. Each chapter is designed to build upon the previous one, guiding you step-by-step from the basics to more advanced techniques and applications.

As you embark on this journey, remember that essential oils are a powerful tool for natural healing and wellness. With the knowledge and resources provided in this book, you will be well-equipped to harness the full potential of essential oils and integrate them into your daily life for improved health, well-being, and overall quality of life.

So, take a deep breath, open your mind, and get ready to unveil the wonders of essential oils. Your path to natural healing and wellness begins here.

Chapter 1: Introduction to Essential Oils

- *What Are Essential Oils?*

- *Common Misconceptions About Essential Oils*

- *Essential Oils in Different Cultures*

- *Integrating Essential Oils into Daily Life*

- *Essential Oil Safety and Precautions*

Essential oils have captivated humanity for centuries, weaving their aromatic and therapeutic magic through various cultures and traditions. In this chapter, we'll explore the essence of these potent plant extracts, debunk common misconceptions, and understand their integration into daily life. We'll also delve into the rich history of essential oils, their diverse cultural significance, and the crucial safety precautions necessary for their effective and safe use.

What Are Essential Oils?

Essential oils are concentrated extracts derived from various parts of plants, including flowers, leaves, bark, roots, and fruits. These oils capture the plant's natural fragrance and beneficial properties, which can be utilized for a range of purposes, from therapeutic applications to culinary uses. The extraction process involves methods such as steam distillation, cold pressing, and solvent extraction, each tailored to preserve the unique characteristics of the plant. We will dive deeper into those methods later on.

The allure of essential oils lies in their potent and multifaceted nature. Unlike synthetic fragrances, essential oils are composed of a complex mixture of organic compounds that can have profound effects on both the mind and body. These compounds include terpenes, esters, alcohols, and aldehydes, among others, each contributing to the oil's distinct aroma and therapeutic properties.

As mentioned in the introduction, essential oils have been used for thousands of years across various cultures for their healing properties. Just to name a few more, in ancient Egypt, oils like frankincense and myrrh were used in religious ceremonies and for embalming. Traditional Chinese and Indian medicine systems, such as Ayurveda, have long incorporated essential oils for their medicinal benefits. We will go over the historical significance of a few more cultures and populations later in the chapter. Modern science has begun to validate many of the traditional uses of essential oils.

The versatility of essential oils extends beyond therapeutic uses. They are commonly used in cosmetics, perfumes, and household cleaning products due to their pleasant scents and natural antibacterial properties. In the culinary world, certain essential oils are used to add flavor and aroma to dishes, providing a concentrated essence of the plant.

To sum up, essential oils are a bridge between the natural world and human well-being. They offer a holistic approach to health, harnessing the power of nature to support physical, emotional, and spiritual wellness. As you delve deeper into the world of essential oils, you will discover a wealth of knowledge and applications that can enhance your life in myriad ways.

Common Misconceptions About Essential Oils

Despite their long history and widespread use, essential oils are often surrounded by myths and misconceptions. These misunderstandings can lead to misuse and unrealistic expectations about their effects. It's important to address and dispel these myths to ensure safe and effective use of essential oils.

One common misconception is that essential oils are completely safe because they are natural. While it's true that essential oils are derived from plants, this does not automatically make them safe for all uses. Essential oils are highly concentrated substances, and improper use can lead to adverse reactions. For instance, applying undiluted essential oils directly to the skin can cause irritation or allergic reactions in some individuals. It's crucial to dilute essential oils with a carrier oil and conduct a patch test before widespread use.

Another myth is that more is better. In the case of essential oils, using larger quantities does not necessarily enhance their benefits. Essential oils are potent, and even a few drops can be effective. Overuse can lead to sensitization, where the body becomes overly reactive to the oil, causing skin irritation or other allergic reactions. It's important to follow recommended dosages and application methods to avoid these issues.

There is also a misconception that essential oils can cure diseases. While essential oils can support overall wellness and alleviate certain symptoms, they are not a substitute for professional medical treatment. Claims that essential oils can cure serious conditions such as cancer or diabetes are not supported by scientific evidence and can be misleading. It's essential to approach essential oils as a complementary therapy, not a primary treatment for medical conditions.

Some people believe that all essential oils are created equal, but the quality of essential oils can vary significantly. Factors such as the plant species, growing conditions, harvesting methods, and extraction processes all influence the final product. Low-quality essential oils may be adulterated with synthetic chemicals or diluted with carrier oils, reducing their effectiveness and safety. It's important to purchase essential oils from reputable sources that provide information about the oil's purity and origin.

Finally, there is a belief that essential oils can be used indiscriminately by everyone. However, certain populations, such as pregnant women, young children, and individuals with specific health conditions, need to use essential oils with caution. For example, some essential oils can affect hormone levels and should be avoided during pregnancy. Always consult with a healthcare provider before using essential oils, especially if you have underlying health concerns.

By addressing these misconceptions, we can promote a more informed and responsible use of essential oils. Understanding their potential and limitations helps users harness their benefits safely and effectively, leading to a more positive and beneficial experience with these powerful natural extracts.

Essential Oils in Different Cultures

Essential oils have played a significant role in various cultures throughout history, each utilizing these potent plant extracts in unique and meaningful ways. From ancient rituals to modern practices, the cultural significance of essential oils spans continents and millennia.

The Egyptians are credited with some of the earliest uses of essential oils, employing them in the embalming process to preserve bodies and prepare them for the afterlife. Oils such as frankincense and myrrh were highly valued, not only for their preservation properties but also for their spiritual significance. Temples often had their own perfumeries, where priests would create blends for rituals and personal use.

As you are aware by now, the ancient Greeks and Romans also embraced the use of essential oils. Greek soldiers would use myrrh to clean and heal battle wounds due to its antiseptic properties. The Romans, on the other hand, were known for their elaborate bathing rituals, where essential oils were used to scent the water, promote relaxation, and enhance overall well-being.

In India, essential oils have been a cornerstone of Ayurvedic medicine for over 3,000 years. Ayurveda, meaning "science of life," incorporates essential oils to balance the body's doshas (biological energies) and promote health and harmony. Oils such as sandalwood, turmeric, and holy basil (tulsi) are commonly used in massage, meditation, and medicinal preparations. Essential oils are also integral to religious ceremonies and daily rituals, reflecting their deep cultural and spiritual importance.

Traditional Chinese Medicine (TCM) has utilized essential oils for centuries as well. In TCM, essential oils are used to address imbalances in the body's qi (life force energy) and to treat various ailments. Oils like ginger and cinnamon are used for their warming properties, while peppermint and eucalyptus are prized for their cooling and invigorating effects. Aromatherapy in TCM often involves inhalation or topical application, combined with other healing modalities like acupuncture and herbal medicine.

Indigenous cultures in the Americas, Australia, and Africa have also long recognized the value of essential oils. Native American tribes used aromatic plants like sage and cedar in smudging rituals to cleanse and purify spaces. Aboriginal Australians utilized tea tree oil for its powerful antiseptic properties, applying it to wounds and skin infections. African cultures often incorporate essential oils into traditional healing practices, using them for their medicinal and aromatic benefits.

In modern times, the global appreciation for essential oils continues to grow, influenced by these rich cultural traditions. The practice of aromatherapy, which uses essential oils to promote physical and emotional well-being, draws on knowledge from various cultures to create a holistic approach to health. Essential oils are now widely used in complementary and alternative medicine, beauty and skincare, and even culinary arts, demonstrating their versatile and enduring appeal.

Understanding the cultural significance of essential oils enriches our appreciation of these natural wonders. By exploring the diverse ways in which different cultures have harnessed the power of essential oils, we can gain a deeper insight into their potential benefits and applications in our own lives.

Integrating Essential Oils into Daily Life

Incorporating essential oils into your daily routine can enhance your physical, emotional, and spiritual well-being. These versatile natural products offer numerous ways to enrich your everyday experiences, from morning rituals to bedtime routines.

Starting your day with essential oils can set a positive tone and boost your energy. Consider adding a few drops of invigorating oils like peppermint or citrus to your morning shower. The steam will disperse the oils, creating a refreshing and energizing atmosphere. Alternatively, you can diffuse these oils in your bathroom or bedroom to help wake up your senses and promote alertness.

For skincare enthusiasts, essential oils can be a valuable addition to your beauty regimen. Oils like lavender and tea tree are known for their skin-soothing properties and can be added to your moisturizer or used in DIY skincare recipes. For a natural glow, consider creating a facial serum by blending essential oils with a carrier oil such as jojoba or argan oil. Remember to always perform a patch test to ensure you don't have an allergic reaction.

During the workday, essential oils can help enhance focus and productivity. Diffusing oils like rosemary, lemon, or eucalyptus in your workspace can improve concentration and mental clarity. If you prefer a more personal touch, create a portable inhaler with your favorite concentration-boosting blend to use throughout the day. Essential oils can also be used in homemade cleaning products, offering a natural and pleasant way to maintain a clean and fresh environment.

Essential oils are also excellent companions for physical exercise. Adding a few drops of eucalyptus or peppermint oil to a damp cloth and inhaling deeply can open your airways and boost your workout performance. After exercise, essential oils like lavender and chamomile can be used in a soothing massage oil to relax muscles and promote recovery.

Incorporating essential oils into your evening routine can help you unwind and prepare for a restful night's sleep. Diffusing calming oils like lavender, cedarwood, or bergamot in your bedroom can create a tranquil atmosphere conducive to relaxation. A warm bath with a few drops of essential oils and Epsom salts can also help soothe tired muscles and calm your mind. For a gentle bedtime ritual, consider applying a diluted blend of relaxing oils to your pulse points or the soles of your feet.

Beyond personal care, essential oils can enhance your culinary experiences. Certain oils, such as lemon, peppermint, and rosemary, can be used in cooking and baking to add concentrated flavor. It's important to use only food-grade essential oils and to add them sparingly, as they are much more potent than dried or fresh herbs.

Lastly, essential oils can play a role in your spiritual practices. They can be used in meditation to create a sacred space and deepen your practice. Frankincense, sandalwood, and patchouli are commonly used for their grounding and centering properties. Whether diffused, inhaled directly, or applied topically, these oils can help you connect with your inner self and promote a sense of peace and balance.

Integrating essential oils into your daily life offers a holistic approach to wellness. By exploring the various ways to incorporate these natural products into your routines, you can discover new levels of enjoyment and benefit from their therapeutic properties. Whether you're looking to boost your energy, enhance your skincare, improve your focus, or relax and unwind, essential oils can be a valuable addition to your lifestyle.

Essential Oil Safety and Precautions

While essential oils offer numerous benefits, it is crucial to use them safely and responsibly. Understanding the potential risks and how to mitigate them is key to enjoying the full advantages of essential oils without adverse effects.

One of the most important safety considerations is dilution. Essential oils are highly concentrated and should never be applied directly to the skin without being diluted in a carrier oil, such as coconut, jojoba, or almond oil. A general guideline is to use a 2% dilution for adults, which equates to about 12 drops of essential oil per ounce of carrier oil. For children, elderly individuals, or those with sensitive skin, a 1% dilution or lower is recommended.

Another critical aspect of essential oil safety is understanding which oils should be avoided during pregnancy, breastfeeding, or by individuals with certain medical conditions. For example, oils like clary sage, rosemary, and cinnamon should be avoided during pregnancy as they can stimulate contractions. Individuals with epilepsy should avoid oils like fennel, sage, and eucalyptus due to their potential to trigger seizures. Always consult with a healthcare provider before using essential oils if you have any underlying health conditions.

Inhalation is a common and generally safe method of using essential oils, but it is still important to exercise caution. Direct inhalation from the bottle or diffuser can be overwhelming and potentially irritating to the respiratory system. It's best to diffuse essential oils in a well-ventilated area and limit exposure to short periods. For those with asthma or other respiratory conditions, certain essential oils can exacerbate symptoms, so it's important to choose oils that are known to be gentle and non-irritating.

Ingestion of essential oils is a highly debated topic. While some practitioners advocate for the internal use of essential oils, it should only be done under the guidance of a qualified healthcare professional. Essential oils are potent substances, and ingesting them without proper knowledge and guidance can lead to toxicity, digestive issues, or interactions with medications.

Storage is another important consideration for maintaining the safety and efficacy of essential oils. Essential oils should be stored in dark glass bottles, away from direct sunlight and heat, to prevent degradation. Proper storage ensures that the oils retain their therapeutic properties and do not become rancid or lose their potency.

It's also important to be aware of potential allergic reactions. Before using a new essential oil, perform a patch test by applying a small amount of diluted oil to the inside of your elbow and waiting 24 hours to check for any adverse reactions. If redness, itching, or irritation occurs, discontinue use immediately.

Lastly, keep essential oils out of reach of children and pets. Some essential oils can be harmful or even toxic to animals. For example, tea tree oil, while beneficial for humans, can be toxic to cats and dogs if ingested or applied to their skin. Always research the safety of essential oils for your specific pets and use them in areas where pets cannot access them.

By adhering to these safety precautions, you can enjoy the many benefits of essential oils while minimizing the risks. Essential oils are powerful tools for enhancing health and well-being, but like all potent substances, they require respectful and informed use. Educating yourself about essential oil safety ensures a positive and beneficial experience, allowing you to fully embrace their healing potential.

Chapter 2: The Extraction and Production of Essential Oils

- *Methods of Extraction: Steam Distillation, Cold Pressing, and Solvent Extraction*

- *The Role of Purity and Quality*

- *Understanding Labels and Certifications*

- *Sustainable Sourcing and Ethical Practices*

- *Home Extraction: DIY Methods*

The journey from plant to bottle involves a meticulous and fascinating process that ensures the purity and potency of essential oils. In this chapter, we will delve into the various methods of extraction, discuss the critical importance of quality and purity, explore the significance of labels and certifications, and highlight the ethical and sustainable practices that underpin responsible production. Additionally, we'll provide insights into DIY extraction methods for those who wish to create their own essential oils at home.

Methods of Extraction: Steam Distillation, Cold Pressing, and Solvent Extraction

The extraction of essential oils from plants is a precise and methodical process that significantly impacts the final product's quality, aroma, and therapeutic properties. The three primary methods of extraction are steam distillation, cold pressing, and solvent extraction, each with its unique advantages and applications.

Steam distillation is the most widely used method for extracting essential oils from plant material. This process involves passing steam through the plant material, which causes the essential oils to vaporize. The steam and oil vapors are then directed into a condenser, where they cool and revert to liquid form. Because essential oils are lighter than water, they naturally separate and can be collected from the top of the distillate. This method is particularly effective for extracting oils from leaves, flowers, and stems, such as lavender, eucalyptus, and rosemary. Steam distillation preserves the integrity of the plant's aromatic compounds, ensuring high-quality essential oils. The temperature and pressure must be carefully controlled to avoid damaging the delicate compounds in the essential oils.

Cold pressing is mainly used for extracting essential oils from citrus fruits, such as oranges, lemons, and grapefruits. This method involves mechanically pressing the rinds or peels of the fruits to release the essential oils. The cold pressing process is purely mechanical and involves no heat, which helps retain the oil's natural aroma and beneficial properties. The pressed oil is then filtered to remove impurities. Cold pressing is valued for producing fresh, vibrant oils that closely resemble the natural scent of the fruit. This method is straightforward and efficient, making it a popular choice for producing citrus oils.

Solvent extraction is employed for delicate plant materials that do not withstand the heat of steam distillation or yield insufficient oil through mechanical methods. This process uses a solvent, such as ethanol or hexane, to dissolve the essential oil from the plant material. The solvent-oil mixture is then filtered, and the solvent is evaporated, leaving behind the concentrated essential oil. Solvent extraction is commonly used for flowers like jasmine and tuberose, producing absolutes— highly concentrated forms of essential oil with intense aromas. While this method can yield a higher amount of oil, it requires careful handling to ensure no harmful solvent residues remain in the final product.

Each extraction method has its advantages and limitations. Steam distillation is ideal for most aromatic plants but may not be suitable for all plant materials. Cold pressing is excellent for citrus oils but limited to specific fruits. Solvent extraction is versatile but requires meticulous processing to ensure safety and purity. Understanding these methods allows consumers and producers to appreciate the complexity involved in producing high-quality essential oils and make informed choices about the products they use.

The Role of Purity and Quality

The purity and quality of essential oils are critical factors that determine their safety, efficacy, and overall value. High-quality essential oils are pure, unadulterated, and free from synthetic additives or contaminants. Achieving such purity begins with the selection of plant material and continues through the extraction and production processes.

Purity refers to the absence of any additional substances in the essential oil. Pure essential oils contain only the natural compounds extracted from the plant, with no synthetic additives, fillers, or diluents. Ensuring purity starts with sourcing high-quality raw materials. Plants must be grown in optimal conditions, harvested at the right time, and processed with care to preserve their essential properties. Any deviation in these factors can affect the oil's purity and therapeutic benefits.

Quality encompasses a broader range of characteristics, including the oil's chemical composition, aroma, color, and therapeutic properties. High-quality essential oils maintain the integrity of the plant's natural compounds, ensuring they deliver the expected benefits. The quality of an essential oil is influenced by various factors, including the plant species, geographical origin, growing conditions, and harvesting methods. For instance, lavender grown in the high altitudes of France's Provence region is known for its superior quality due to the ideal climate and soil conditions.

To assess the quality of essential oils, **gas chromatography-mass spectrometry (GC-MS)** is often used. This analytical technique identifies the chemical constituents of the oil and their concentrations, providing a detailed profile of its composition. GC-MS testing helps verify the authenticity and purity of the oil, ensuring that it meets industry standards and consumer expectations. Reputable producers conduct regular GC-MS testing to maintain quality control and provide transparency to their customers.

Certifications and labels also play a crucial role in indicating the quality and purity of essential oils.

Certifications like USDA Organic, ISO (International Organization for Standardization), and EOBBD (Essential Oil Botanically and Biochemically Defined) offer assurance that the oils have been produced according to stringent standards. Organic certification, for example, guarantees that the plants were grown without synthetic pesticides or fertilizers, contributing to the purity and sustainability of the oil.

Consumers should seek out reputable suppliers who provide detailed information about their sourcing, extraction methods, and quality assurance practices. By choosing high-quality essential oils, individuals can enjoy the full benefits of these natural products with confidence in their safety and efficacy.

Understanding Labels and Certifications

Navigating the world of essential oils can be challenging, especially when it comes to understanding labels and certifications. These elements provide vital information about the product's quality, purity, and sourcing, helping consumers make informed choices.

Labels on essential oil bottles should provide key details about the product. A high-quality essential oil label typically includes the following information:

1. **Botanical Name**: The Latin name of the plant from which the oil is extracted. This ensures clarity and avoids confusion, as common names can vary between regions and brands. For example, "Lavandula angustifolia" specifies true lavender, while "Lavandula latifolia" refers to spike lavender, which has different properties.

2. **Part of Plant Used**: This indicates which part of the plant was used to extract the oil, such as leaves, flowers, bark, or roots. Different parts of the same plant can yield oils with distinct properties.

3. **Method of Extraction**: This details how the oil was extracted, such as steam distillation, cold pressing, or

solvent extraction. Knowing the extraction method helps understand the purity and potential uses of the oil.

4. **Country of Origin**: The geographical source of the plant can influence the oil's quality. Certain regions are renowned for producing high-quality essential oils due to their climate, soil, and traditional farming practices.

5. **Batch Number**: This allows traceability back to the specific batch of oil, which is useful for quality control and addressing any issues that may arise.

6. **Expiration Date**: Essential oils can degrade over time, losing their potency and therapeutic benefits. An expiration date ensures the oil is used within its optimal period.

Certifications provide additional assurance about the quality and ethical standards of essential oils. Key certifications to look for include:

1. **USDA Organic**: Indicates that the oil is derived from plants grown without synthetic pesticides, herbicides, or genetically modified organisms (GMOs). Organic certification also implies sustainable farming practices that protect the environment.

2. **ISO (International Organization for Standardization)**: ISO standards for essential oils ensure consistency, purity, and quality across different batches. ISO certification means the oil meets internationally recognized standards for its chemical composition and production methods.

3. **EOBBD (Essential Oil Botanically and Biochemically Defined)**: This certification ensures that the essential oil is authentic and unadulterated, with a defined chemical profile that matches the expected properties of the plant species.

4. **Fair Trade**: Fair Trade certification indicates that the essential oil was produced under ethical labor practices, ensuring fair wages and working conditions for farmers and workers.

5. **Cruelty-Free**: This label signifies that the product and its ingredients were not tested on animals, aligning with ethical and humane standards.

Understanding labels and certifications helps consumers select essential oils that meet their quality and ethical expectations. By paying attention to these details, individuals can ensure they are purchasing products that are pure, effective, and produced in a manner that respects both people and the planet.

Sustainable Sourcing and Ethical Practices

The increasing demand for essential oils has brought attention to the importance of sustainable sourcing and ethical practices in their production. Sustainable sourcing ensures that the harvesting of plants for essential oils does not harm the environment or deplete natural resources, while ethical practices prioritize the well-being of workers and communities involved in the production process.

Sustainable sourcing begins with responsible cultivation and harvesting practices. Plants used for essential oils should be grown without harmful pesticides or synthetic fertilizers, which can damage ecosystems and contaminate water supplies. Organic farming methods, crop rotation, and intercropping are techniques that promote soil health and biodiversity, ensuring the long-term sustainability of plant resources.

Harvesting practices also play a crucial role in sustainability. For example, wild-harvested plants must be collected in a way that allows the population to regenerate. Over-harvesting can lead to the depletion of plant species and disrupt local ecosystems. Sustainable harvesting involves careful planning and monitoring to ensure that only a portion of the plants are collected, leaving enough to reproduce and maintain the ecological balance.

Ethical practices in essential oil production extend beyond environmental considerations to encompass the fair treatment of workers and communities. Fair Trade certification is one way to ensure that farmers and workers receive fair wages and work in safe conditions. This certification also often includes community development initiatives, such as funding for schools, healthcare, and infrastructure, which benefit the entire community.

Transparent supply chains are another aspect of ethical practices. Consumers should be able to trace the origin of their essential oils and verify that they are sourced from reputable suppliers who adhere to ethical standards. This transparency helps build trust and accountability in the industry.

In addition to fair wages and working conditions, ethical practices involve respecting the cultural heritage and traditional knowledge of indigenous communities who have been using aromatic plants for centuries. Companies should engage with these communities in a way that honors their traditions and shares the benefits of commercializing their traditional plants. This can include profit-sharing agreements, investing in local infrastructure, and ensuring that the community has a say in how their natural resources are used.

Certification programs play a vital role in promoting sustainable and ethical practices. Certifications such as USDA Organic, Fair Trade, and Rainforest Alliance provide third-party verification that essential oils are produced in accordance with rigorous environmental and social standards. These certifications help consumers identify products that align with their values and support sustainable and ethical production methods.

Home Extraction: DIY Methods

For those who enjoy hands-on projects and want to control the quality and purity of their essential oils, home extraction can be an appealing option. While commercial extraction methods like steam distillation and cold pressing require specialized equipment, there are simpler DIY methods that can be done at home using readily available materials.

Steam Distillation: While true steam distillation requires specialized equipment, a simplified version can be done at home using a pot, a heat-resistant bowl, and ice. To extract essential oils using this method, place the plant material in a large pot with water. Place a heat-resistant bowl on top of the plant material but make sure it does not touch the water. Cover the pot with an inverted lid filled with ice. As the water heats up and produces steam, the steam will rise, carrying the essential oil vapors. The vapors will condense when they hit the cold lid and drip into the bowl. This DIY setup mimics the basic principles of steam distillation, although it may not be as efficient or yield as pure a product as professional equipment.

Infusion and Maceration: These methods are suitable for extracting oils from herbs and flowers. Infusion involves soaking plant material in a carrier oil, such as olive or coconut oil, and heating it gently to release the essential oils into the carrier oil. The mixture is then strained to remove the plant material, leaving behind a fragrant infused oil. Maceration is similar but involves crushing or bruising the plant material to help release the oils before soaking it in the carrier oil. These methods are relatively simple and can be done with basic kitchen equipment.

Cold Pressing: While true cold pressing requires heavy machinery, a modified version can be done at home for small-scale extraction, especially for citrus oils. Simply grate the citrus peels to release the oils and then use a heavy object, such as a rolling pin, to press the grated peels over a piece of cheesecloth. Squeeze the cheesecloth to extract the oil. This method is labor-intensive and yields a small amount of oil, but it can be a fun and educational project.

Alcohol Extraction: This method uses high-proof alcohol to extract essential oils from plant material. Place the plant material in a jar and cover it with alcohol. Let it sit for several days, shaking the jar occasionally. The alcohol will dissolve the essential oils from the plant material. After the extraction period, strain out the plant material and allow the alcohol to evaporate, leaving behind the essential oil. This method can be effective but requires patience and proper ventilation to handle the evaporating alcohol.

While home extraction methods can be rewarding and provide a sense of accomplishment, they also come with limitations. The yield is typically lower, and the purity and concentration of the oils may not match commercially produced essential oils. However, these methods offer a hands-on way to explore the world of essential oils and create custom blends for personal use. Always use caution and follow safety guidelines when attempting home extraction to ensure the best results and avoid any potential hazards.

Home extraction of essential oils can be a fascinating hobby that provides insight into the complexities of essential oil production. It allows enthusiasts to experiment with different plants and methods, gaining a deeper appreciation for the art and science behind these aromatic substances.

Chapter 3: Popular Oils and Their Properties

- *Lavender: The Calming Healer*

- *Peppermint: The Energizing Coolant*

- *Eucalyptus: The Respiratory Aid*

- *Tea Tree: The Antimicrobial Warrior*

- *Lemon: The Uplifting Cleanser*

In this chapter, we'll explore five popular essential oils known for their unique properties and diverse range of uses in wellness practices. Their popularity also stems from their natural origins, offering holistic solutions that align with the growing interest in natural and alternative therapies.

Lavender: The Calming Healer

Lavender essential oil, extracted from Lavandula angustifolia flowers, is renowned for its calming and soothing properties. Its use dates back thousands of years, with ancient civilizations such as the Egyptians and Romans using it for bathing, relaxation, and as a perfume.

One of the key components of lavender oil is linalool, which has been extensively studied for its effects on the nervous system. Research suggests that inhaling lavender oil can reduce anxiety and improve mood by interacting with neurotransmitters in the brain. Its calming effects are why it's often used in aromatherapy to promote relaxation and improve sleep quality.

In addition to its psychological benefits, lavender oil also offers physical health benefits. It has anti-inflammatory and antimicrobial properties, making it effective for treating minor burns, wounds, and insect bites. It can also help alleviate symptoms of conditions like eczema and acne.

To use lavender oil, you can add a few drops to a diffuser to enjoy its calming aroma, dilute it with a carrier oil for a relaxing massage, or add it to your bath for a soothing soak. It's generally safe for most people when used topically or aromatically, but it's essential to do a patch test first and consult with a healthcare professional if you have any concerns.

Peppermint: The Energizing Coolant

Peppermint essential oil, derived from Mentha piperita leaves, is known for its invigorating and refreshing properties. Its minty aroma is instantly recognizable and has a cooling effect on the skin and senses.

One of the main components of peppermint oil is menthol, which gives it its characteristic cooling sensation. Menthol has analgesic properties, making peppermint oil effective for relieving headaches, muscle aches, and itching. It's also a natural decongestant, making it useful for clearing sinuses and relieving symptoms of colds and allergies.

Peppermint oil is also known for its ability to improve mental clarity and focus. Studies have shown that inhaling peppermint oil can enhance memory and alertness, making it a popular choice for studying or working.

To use peppermint oil, you can inhale it directly from the bottle, add a few drops to a diffuser, or dilute it with a carrier oil for topical use. It's important to note that peppermint oil is potent and should be used sparingly, especially around children and pregnant women. Always dilute it before applying it to the skin and avoid contact with sensitive areas like the eyes.

Eucalyptus: The Respiratory Aid

Eucalyptus essential oil, extracted from the leaves of eucalyptus trees, is well-known for its respiratory benefits. It has a fresh, camphoraceous aroma that is both invigorating and clarifying.

One of the primary components of eucalyptus oil is 1,8-cineole, also known as eucalyptol, which has been extensively studied for its effects on the respiratory system. It has mucolytic properties, meaning it can help break down mucus and phlegm, making it easier to expel. This makes eucalyptus oil effective for relieving symptoms of respiratory conditions such as colds, flu, and bronchitis.

In addition to its respiratory benefits, eucalyptus oil also has antimicrobial properties, making it useful for treating wounds, cuts, and insect bites. It can also be used as a natural insect repellent.

To use eucalyptus oil, you can inhale it directly from the bottle, add a few drops to a bowl of hot water and inhale the steam, or dilute it with a carrier oil and apply it to the chest or back for respiratory relief. As with all essential oils, it's essential to dilute eucalyptus oil before applying it to the skin and avoid contact with sensitive areas.

Tea Tree: The Antimicrobial Warrior

Tea tree essential oil, also known as melaleuca oil, is extracted from the leaves of the tea tree (Melaleuca alternifolia). It has a fresh, medicinal scent and is well-known for its powerful antimicrobial properties.

One of the main active components of tea tree oil is terpinen-4-ol, which has been shown to have broad-spectrum antimicrobial activity against bacteria, viruses, and fungi. This makes tea tree oil a popular choice for treating various skin conditions, including acne, fungal infections, and insect bites.

Tea tree oil is also known for its anti-inflammatory properties, making it effective for reducing redness and swelling associated with skin inflammation. It can also help soothe itching and irritation.

To use tea tree oil, you can dilute it with a carrier oil and apply it to the skin, add a few drops to a warm bath, or mix it with water in a spray bottle for a natural household cleaner. It's important to note that tea tree oil can cause skin irritation in some people, so it's essential to do a patch test before using it extensively.

Lemon: The Uplifting Cleanser

Lemon essential oil, extracted from the peel of fresh lemons (Citrus limon), has a bright, citrusy aroma that is uplifting and energizing. It's known for its cleansing and purifying properties, both for the body and the environment.

One of the main components of lemon oil is limonene, which has been studied for its mood-enhancing effects. Inhaling lemon oil can help improve mood and reduce feelings of stress and anxiety. Its refreshing scent can also help increase focus and concentration.

Lemon oil is also a potent antimicrobial agent, making it an excellent natural cleaner. It can help disinfect surfaces and freshen the air. Additionally, lemon oil can be used in skincare to help reduce excess oil and improve the appearance of skin tone and texture.

To use lemon oil, you can add a few drops to a diffuser to enjoy its uplifting aroma, dilute it with a carrier oil for a refreshing massage, or add it to your cleaning products for a natural disinfectant. It's important to note that lemon oil can cause photosensitivity, so it's essential to avoid direct sunlight after topical application.

These popular essential oils offer a range of benefits for both physical and emotional well-being, making them valuable additions to any natural health and wellness routine.

Chapter 4: Aromatherapy & the Art of Using Essential Oils

- *What is Aromatherapy?*

- *Benefits of Aromatherapy*

- *Techniques: Diffusion, Inhalation, and Topical Application*

- *Creating Your Own Aromatherapy Blends*

- *Aromatherapy for Emotional Wellness*

Aromatherapy is a holistic healing treatment that utilizes natural plant extracts, known as essential oils, to promote health and well-being. These potent oils are extracted from various parts of plants, including flowers, leaves, stems, bark, and roots, using methods like steam distillation or cold pressing. Each essential oil carries its own unique aroma and therapeutic properties, which are believed to offer numerous benefits to the body, mind, and spirit.

What is Aromatherapy?

Aromatherapy, also referred to as essential oil therapy, is a therapeutic approach that harnesses the aromatic compounds of plants for healing purposes. This practice dates back thousands of years and has been used by ancient civilizations such as the Egyptians, Greeks, and Romans for its medicinal and spiritual benefits. Today, aromatherapy is recognized as a complementary therapy that can support conventional medical treatments.

Essential oils are highly concentrated extracts obtained from plants. They contain volatile compounds that give them their characteristic aroma and therapeutic properties. These oils can be used in various ways, including inhalation, topical application, and in some cases, ingestion (although ingestion should only be done under the guidance of a qualified practitioner due to safety concerns).

Aromatherapy is based on the notion that aromatic compounds in essential oils can influence the physical, emotional, and psychological aspects of well-being. When inhaled, the molecules in essential oils travel through the olfactory system, which is connected to the brain's limbic system. The limbic system is responsible for controlling emotions, memories, and arousal. This connection allows the scent of essential oils to have a direct impact on emotional responses and mood regulation.

Additionally, essential oils can be absorbed through the skin and enter the bloodstream, where they can exert their therapeutic effects throughout the body. The use of carrier oils, such as jojoba, coconut, or almond oil, is crucial in diluting essential oils for safe topical application. Carrier oils not only help in the absorption of essential oils but also provide their own moisturizing and nourishing benefits to the skin.

Aromatherapy can be incorporated into a variety of wellness practices, including massages, baths, and skincare routines. It is commonly used in spa treatments to enhance relaxation and rejuvenation. Many holistic practitioners integrate aromatherapy into their treatment protocols to complement other therapies, such as massage therapy, acupuncture, and chiropractic care.

Moreover, aromatherapy is often used in conjunction with meditation and yoga practices to enhance mental clarity, focus, and spiritual connection. By creating a serene and calming environment, essential oils can support mindfulness and deepen the overall experience of these practices.

Research into the efficacy of aromatherapy has shown

promising results, particularly in the areas of stress reduction, pain management, and improved sleep quality. Studies have demonstrated that certain essential oils can influence the autonomic nervous system, promoting relaxation and reducing stress hormones like cortisol. This makes aromatherapy a valuable tool for managing anxiety and enhancing emotional resilience.

Furthermore, the antimicrobial properties of some essential oils have been recognized for their potential to fight infections and support the immune system. Oils like tea tree, eucalyptus, and thyme have been found to exhibit antibacterial, antiviral, and antifungal effects, making them useful for preventing and treating minor infections.

Aromatherapy is also increasingly being explored in clinical settings for its potential benefits in palliative care and chronic illness management. Essential oils can provide comfort and improve the quality of life for patients by alleviating symptoms such as pain, nausea, and anxiety. In hospice care, aromatherapy is used to create a soothing atmosphere and provide emotional support to patients and their families.

Despite its many benefits, it is important to approach aromatherapy with a sense of caution and respect for the potency of essential oils. Proper dilution and usage guidelines must be followed to avoid adverse reactions, and it is always recommended to consult with a qualified aromatherapist or healthcare professional, especially when using essential oils for medical purposes.

In summary, aromatherapy is a versatile and accessible form of holistic therapy that harnesses the power of plant-derived essential oils to promote physical, emotional, and psychological well-being. Its rich history and growing body of scientific research underscore its value as a complementary therapy that can enhance overall health and quality of life.

Benefits of Aromatherapy

Aromatherapy has gained significant popularity as a natural and effective method for stress relief. This therapeutic practice uses essential oils to promote relaxation, reduce anxiety, and improve overall emotional well-being. The following detailed points explain why aromatherapy is particularly beneficial for stress relief:

1. Direct Impact on the Limbic System: The olfactory system, responsible for our sense of smell, is directly connected to the limbic system in the brain. The limbic system controls emotions, memories, and behaviors. When we inhale the aroma of essential oils, the molecules stimulate olfactory receptors, which send signals to the brain, specifically the limbic system. This interaction can trigger emotional responses and help regulate mood, making aromatherapy an effective tool for managing stress.

2. Neurochemical Release: Inhaling certain essential oils can stimulate the release of neurotransmitters such as serotonin and dopamine. These chemicals play a crucial role in mood regulation and can induce feelings of happiness and relaxation. For instance, lavender oil has been shown to increase serotonin levels, which helps alleviate stress and anxiety.

3. Cortisol Reduction: Cortisol, known as the stress hormone, is released in response to stress and can have negative effects on the body if levels remain elevated for prolonged periods. Studies have demonstrated that essential oils like bergamot and lavender can reduce cortisol levels in the body. Lowering cortisol levels helps mitigate the physical and emotional effects of stress, leading to a more relaxed state.

4. Relaxation of the Nervous System: Certain essential oils possess sedative properties that can calm the nervous system. Oils such as chamomile, ylang-ylang, and sandalwood are known for their ability to promote relaxation and reduce nervous tension. When used in aromatherapy, these oils can help soothe the mind and body, providing a sense of tranquility and calmness.

5. Improved Sleep Quality: Stress often disrupts sleep patterns, leading to insomnia or poor-quality sleep. Essential oils like lavender, valerian, and cedarwood have been widely used to improve sleep quality. By promoting relaxation and reducing anxiety, these oils can help individuals fall asleep faster and enjoy deeper, more restorative sleep, which is essential for managing stress effectively.

6. Enhanced Breathing and Respiratory Function: Stress can cause shallow breathing or hyperventilation, exacerbating feelings of anxiety. Essential oils such as eucalyptus, peppermint, and rosemary can support respiratory function by opening airways and improving breathing. When inhaled, these oils can help individuals take deeper, more calming breaths, which can significantly reduce stress levels.

7. Creation of a Calming Environment: Diffusing essential oils in living spaces can create a calming and serene atmosphere. This environmental enhancement can provide a sense of safety and comfort, making it easier to relax and unwind. Oils like frankincense and sandalwood are particularly effective in creating a peaceful environment conducive to relaxation and stress relief.

8. Synergistic Effects with Other Relaxation Techniques: Aromatherapy can be combined with other relaxation techniques, such as meditation, yoga, and massage, to enhance their stress-relieving effects. For example, using essential oils during a massage can amplify the relaxation experience by soothing muscles and calming the mind simultaneously. Similarly, diffusing calming oils during meditation or yoga can deepen the practice and promote a more profound sense of relaxation.

9. Personal Empowerment and Self-Care: Engaging in aromatherapy practices can empower individuals to take an active role in their own stress management. Creating personalized blends, choosing favorite scents, and incorporating aromatherapy into daily routines can foster a sense of control and self-care. This proactive approach to stress relief can improve overall emotional resilience and well-being.

10. Accessibility and Versatility: Aromatherapy is accessible and versatile, making it an easy and convenient option for stress relief. Essential oils can be used in various forms, such as diffusers, inhalers, baths, and topical applications, allowing individuals to integrate aromatherapy into their lives in ways that best suit their preferences and needs.

In conclusion, aromatherapy offers a multifaceted

approach to stress relief by leveraging the powerful connection between scent and emotion. Through its direct impact on the brain, modulation of neurochemicals, and creation of a calming environment, aromatherapy provides a natural and effective means of managing stress and enhancing overall emotional well-being. Whether used alone or in combination with other relaxation techniques, essential oils can play a valuable role in promoting relaxation and reducing the negative effects of stress.

Techniques: Diffusion, Inhalation, and Topical Application

Aromatherapy involves various techniques to utilize the benefits of essential oils. Each method offers unique advantages and requires specific application methods to ensure safety and effectiveness. Here are detailed descriptions of the primary techniques used in aromatherapy:

Diffusion

How to Do It: Diffusion involves dispersing essential oils into the air, allowing their aromatic molecules to be inhaled. There are several types of diffusers available:

- **Ultrasonic Diffusers:** These use ultrasonic waves to

create a fine mist of water and essential oils. Simply fill the diffuser with water, add a few drops of essential oil, and turn it on. Ultrasonic diffusers are quiet and often double as humidifiers.

- **Nebulizing Diffusers:** These break down essential oils into tiny particles without using water or heat. They are highly effective for delivering a potent aroma but tend to be more expensive.

- **Evaporative Diffusers:** These use a fan to blow air through a pad or filter containing essential oils. While not as powerful as nebulizing diffusers, they are more affordable and portable.

- **Heat Diffusers:** These use heat to evaporate essential oils. While easy to use, heat can alter the chemical composition of some essential oils, potentially reducing their therapeutic benefits.

Benefits:

- **Air Purification:** Diffusing essential oils like eucalyptus, tea tree, and lemon can help purify the air by reducing airborne pathogens and allergens.

- **Mood Enhancement:** Citrus oils such as orange and grapefruit can uplift the mood, while lavender and chamomile promote relaxation and reduce stress.

- **Respiratory Support:** Oils like peppermint and eucalyptus can help clear nasal passages and support respiratory health.

Health Concerns and Cautions:

- **Overexposure:** Continuous diffusion can lead to headaches, nausea, or sensitization. It's recommended to diffuse essential oils for 30-60 minutes at a time.

- **Pets and Children:** Some essential oils can be harmful to pets and children. Ensure good ventilation and use pet- and child-safe oils when diffusing in shared spaces.

- **Quality of Oils:** Use high-quality, pure essential oils to avoid inhaling potentially harmful additives or contaminants.

Inhalation

How to Do It: Inhalation involves directly breathing in the aroma of essential oils. This method can be simple and immediate:

- **Steam Inhalation:** Add a few drops of essential oil to

a bowl of hot water. Cover your head with a towel and inhale the steam deeply for several minutes. This method is particularly effective for respiratory issues.

- **Aromatherapy Inhalers:** These small, portable devices contain a wick soaked in essential oil. Inhale directly from the inhaler whenever needed for a quick dose of aromatherapy.

- **Direct Inhalation:** Simply open a bottle of essential oil and inhale the aroma directly. Alternatively, place a few drops on a tissue or cotton ball and inhale.

Benefits:

- **Rapid Effect:** Inhalation allows essential oils to quickly enter the bloodstream via the lungs, providing fast relief for conditions like stress, anxiety, and respiratory congestion.

- **Ease of Use:** Inhalation is straightforward and can be done anywhere, making it a convenient option for immediate stress relief or mental clarity.

Health Concerns and Cautions:

- **Irritation:** Some essential oils can be irritating to the mucous membranes. Avoid using oils like cinnamon and clove for direct inhalation.

- **Asthma and Allergies:** Individuals with asthma or allergies should exercise caution, as some essential oils can trigger symptoms.

- **Prolonged Use:** Avoid continuous inhalation over long periods to prevent sensitization or adverse reactions.

Topical Application

How to Do It: Topical application involves applying essential oils directly to the skin. Due to their potency, essential oils should always be diluted with a carrier oil:

- **Dilution:** Mix essential oils with a carrier oil (e.g., jojoba, coconut, almond oil) to create a safe and effective blend. Common dilution ratios are 2-3 drops of essential oil per teaspoon of carrier oil for general use.

- **Massage:** Use diluted essential oils during massage to relieve muscle tension, enhance circulation, and promote relaxation. Apply the blend to sore muscles or joints and massage gently.

- **Skincare:** Incorporate essential oils into your skincare routine by adding a few drops to lotions, creams, or facial oils. This can help with issues like acne, aging, and dryness.

- **Baths:** Add diluted essential oils to bathwater for a relaxing and therapeutic soak. Ensure the oils are mixed with a carrier oil or a dispersant like Epsom salts to prevent skin irritation.

Benefits:

- **Targeted Relief:** Topical application allows for localized treatment of pain, inflammation, and skin conditions.

- **Skin Health:** Essential oils like tea tree, lavender, and frankincense can improve skin health and address issues such as acne, eczema, and aging.

Health Concerns and Cautions:

- **Skin Sensitization:** Some essential oils can cause skin irritation or allergic reactions. Always perform a patch test by applying a small amount of the diluted oil to a patch of skin and observing for any adverse reactions over 24 hours.

- **Photosensitivity:** Citrus oils like lemon, lime, and

bergamot can cause photosensitivity, leading to skin burns or pigmentation when exposed to sunlight. Avoid sun exposure after applying these oils.

- **Proper Dilution:** Undiluted essential oils can be too harsh for the skin and cause irritation or burns. Always dilute essential oils before applying them to the skin.

Internal Use (Caution)

How to Do It: Internal use of essential oils involves consuming them orally. This method should only be done under the guidance of a qualified healthcare practitioner due to the potential risks and interactions with medications.

- **Capsules:** Essential oils can be encapsulated and taken as supplements for specific health issues.

- **Food and Beverages:** Some essential oils can be added to food or drinks for flavor and therapeutic benefits.

Benefits:

- **Systemic Support:** Internal use can provide systemic support for digestive issues, immune function, and overall health.

Health Concerns and Cautions:

- **Toxicity:** Some essential oils can be toxic when ingested, even in small amounts. Oils like wintergreen, eucalyptus, and tea tree should never be taken internally.

- **Interactions:** Essential oils can interact with medications and other supplements. Always consult with a healthcare provider before using essential oils internally.

- **Quality and Purity:** Ensure the essential oils used for internal consumption are of the highest quality and labeled as safe for ingestion.

In conclusion, aromatherapy offers various techniques to harness the benefits of essential oils, each with its own set of advantages and precautions. Whether diffusing, inhaling, or applying topically, understanding the proper methods and safety considerations is crucial to maximizing the therapeutic effects of essential oils while minimizing potential risks..

Creating Your Own Aromatherapy Blends

Creating personalized aromatherapy blends can be a rewarding and therapeutic endeavor. The process involves selecting essential oils based on their therapeutic properties, combining them to achieve a desired effect, and experimenting with different ratios to create a harmonious blend. Here's a detailed guide on how to create and personalize your own aromatherapy blends:

Step 1: Define Your Purpose

The first step in creating an aromatherapy blend is to determine the purpose of the blend. Understanding why you want to create the blend will guide your choice of essential oils. Common purposes include:

- **Relaxation and Stress Relief:** Blends designed to promote relaxation and reduce stress often include calming oils.

- **Energy and Upliftment:** Blends that energize and uplift typically feature invigorating oils.

- **Focus and Concentration:** Blends for mental clarity and focus use oils that enhance cognitive function.

- **Sleep Aid:** Blends to improve sleep quality use sedative and soothing oils.

- **Pain Relief:** Blends for pain relief incorporate oils with analgesic and anti-inflammatory properties.

- **Immune Support:** Blends designed to boost the immune system use oils with antimicrobial and immune-stimulating properties.

Step 2: Choosing Your Essential Oils

Once you have defined the purpose of your blend, the next step is to choose the essential oils that will best achieve your desired outcome. Here are some common essential oils and their therapeutic properties:

Relaxation and Stress Relief

- **Lavender:** Known for its calming and soothing properties, lavender is excellent for reducing anxiety and promoting relaxation.

- **Chamomile:** This gentle oil is effective for calming the mind and alleviating stress.

- **Frankincense:** Frankincense is grounding and can help reduce feelings of anxiety and promote a sense of peace.

Energy and Upliftment

- **Peppermint:** Peppermint oil is invigorating and helps improve mental clarity and energy levels.

- **Lemon:** This citrus oil is uplifting and can enhance mood and increase energy.

- **Eucalyptus:** Eucalyptus is refreshing and can help clear the mind, making it great for an energy boost.

Focus and Concentration

- **Rosemary:** Rosemary oil is known for its ability to enhance memory and concentration.

- **Basil:** This oil supports mental clarity and focus.

- **Cedarwood:** Cedarwood is grounding and can help improve concentration and mental acuity.

Sleep Aid

- **Lavender:** Its sedative properties make it ideal for promoting restful sleep.

- **Valerian:** Valerian oil is a powerful sleep aid and can help with insomnia.

- **Sandalwood:** This oil is soothing and helps calm the mind, promoting better sleep.

Pain Relief

- **Peppermint:** Its analgesic properties make it effective for relieving headaches and muscle pain.

- **Eucalyptus:** Eucalyptus oil is anti-inflammatory and can help reduce pain and swelling.

- **Ginger:** Ginger oil is warming and can help with muscle aches and joint pain.

Immune Support

- **Tea Tree:** Known for its antimicrobial properties, tea tree oil can help boost the immune system.

- **Thyme:** Thyme oil is a powerful immune stimulant and has antiviral properties.

- **Oregano:** Oregano oil is highly antimicrobial and supports the immune system.

Step 3: Experiment with Ratios and Notes

When creating a blend, it's important to consider the different "notes" of the essential oils you're using. These are categorized into top, middle, and base notes based on their evaporation rates and aromatic profiles.

- **Top Notes:** These oils evaporate quickly and provide the initial impression of the blend. Examples include citrus oils (e.g., lemon, orange) and some mints (e.g., peppermint).

- **Middle Notes:** These oils form the body of the blend and have a moderate evaporation rate. Examples include lavender, rosemary, and chamomile.

- **Base Notes:** These oils evaporate slowly and add depth and grounding to the blend. Examples include frankincense, sandalwood, and cedarwood.

A balanced blend typically includes oils from each category to create a harmonious and long-lasting aroma.

Step 4: Creating the Blend

1. **Start Small:** Begin with small quantities to test the blend. A typical ratio is 3-5 drops of essential oil per 1 teaspoon of carrier oil for topical applications.

2. **Use a Dropper:** Use a dropper to accurately measure the essential oils. Start with fewer drops, as you can always add more if needed.

3. **Mix the Oils:** In a small glass bottle or vial, add the essential oils one at a time, starting with the base notes, followed by the middle notes, and finishing with the top notes.

4. **Dilute with Carrier Oil:** If you're making a blend for topical application, dilute the essential oils with a carrier oil. Popular carrier oils include jojoba, sweet almond, coconut, and grapeseed oil.

Step 5: Test and Adjust

After creating your blend, it's important to test it:

1. **Patch Test:** Apply a small amount of the blend to a patch of skin (like the inside of your wrist) to check for any allergic reactions or sensitivities. Wait 24 hours to ensure there is no adverse reaction.

2. **Smell Test:** Allow the blend to rest for a few hours or overnight, then smell it to see how the aromas have melded together. If necessary, adjust the blend by adding more of certain oils to achieve the desired scent.

Step 6: Store Properly

Store your aromatherapy blend in a dark glass bottle to protect it from light, which can degrade the essential oils. Label the bottle with the date and the ingredients used. Keep the blend in a cool, dark place to maintain its potency and shelf life.

Health Concerns and Cautions

Creating and using aromatherapy blends safely is crucial:

- **Proper Dilution:** Essential oils are highly concentrated and should always be diluted with a carrier oil before topical application to avoid skin irritation or sensitization.

- **Patch Testing:** Always perform a patch test with a new blend to check for allergic reactions.

- **Avoiding Certain Oils:** Some essential oils are not recommended for use during pregnancy, for young children, or for individuals with certain medical conditions. Research or consult a qualified aromatherapist before using oils in these cases.

- **Photosensitivity:** Be cautious with citrus oils, as they can cause photosensitivity and increase the risk of skin burns or pigmentation when exposed to sunlight.

- **Quality of Oils:** Use high-quality, pure essential oils from reputable sources to avoid contaminants and adulterants that can be harmful.

In conclusion, creating personalized aromatherapy blends is a creative and therapeutic process that allows you to tailor the benefits of essential oils to your specific needs. By understanding the properties of different oils, experimenting with ratios, and following safety guidelines, you can craft effective and enjoyable aromatherapy blends for various purposes.

Aromatherapy for Emotional Wellness

Aromatherapy can profoundly influence emotional well-being by leveraging the powerful connection between scent and emotion. This connection is rooted in the anatomy and function of the olfactory system and the brain's limbic system. Here's a detailed look at how aromatherapy impacts emotional wellness and how incorporating it into daily practice can enhance overall health and well-being.

The Science Behind Scent and Emotion

1. The Olfactory System: The olfactory system is responsible for our sense of smell and is closely linked to the brain's limbic system, which controls emotions, memories, and behavior. When we inhale an aroma, the scent molecules stimulate olfactory receptors in the nose, sending signals directly to the limbic system. This unique pathway allows scents to elicit immediate emotional and physiological responses.

2. Limbic System and Emotions: The limbic system includes structures such as the hippocampus, amygdala, and hypothalamus, which play crucial roles in regulating emotions, mood, and memory. Aromas can trigger the release of neurotransmitters like serotonin, dopamine, and endorphins, which influence mood and emotional states.

For example, the scent of lavender can promote relaxation and reduce anxiety by stimulating the release of serotonin.

Benefits of Aromatherapy for Emotional Wellness

1. Stress Reduction: Essential oils such as lavender, bergamot, and ylang-ylang are known for their calming properties. They can help lower cortisol levels, the hormone associated with stress, and promote a sense of calm and relaxation.

2. Mood Enhancement: Citrus oils like orange, lemon, and grapefruit are uplifting and energizing. They can help alleviate symptoms of depression, boost mood, and increase feelings of happiness and well-being.

3. Anxiety Relief: Oils such as chamomile, frankincense, and sandalwood have grounding properties that can help reduce anxiety and promote emotional stability. Inhalation of these oils can calm the mind and reduce anxious thoughts.

4. Improved Sleep: Essential oils like lavender, valerian, and cedarwood can promote better sleep quality by inducing relaxation and reducing insomnia. A good night's sleep is essential for emotional resilience and overall well-being.

5. Enhanced Focus and Concentration: Oils like rosemary, peppermint, and basil can enhance cognitive function, improve focus, and support mental clarity. This can be particularly beneficial for individuals experiencing stress or anxiety that impacts their ability to concentrate.

Daily Practice of Aromatherapy

1. Morning Ritual: Start your day by diffusing energizing oils like lemon or peppermint to boost energy levels and enhance mood. This can help set a positive tone for the day ahead.

2. Workplace Aromatherapy: Use a personal inhaler or a small diffuser with oils like rosemary or basil at your workspace to improve focus and concentration. This can enhance productivity and reduce work-related stress.

3. Midday Stress Relief: Take short breaks during the day to practice deep breathing with calming oils like lavender or chamomile. This can help manage stress levels and maintain emotional balance.

4. Evening Wind-Down: Create a relaxing evening routine by diffusing calming oils like lavender or sandalwood. Incorporate these oils into a warm bath or use them in a massage to unwind and prepare for restful sleep.

5. Bedtime Routine: Apply a diluted blend of sleep-promoting oils like cedarwood or valerian to your wrists or pillow before bed. This can help signal to your body that it's time to relax and sleep.

To Surmise

Aromatherapy is a natural and versatile approach to enhancing health and well-being, offering profound benefits for emotional wellness. By leveraging the powerful connection between scent and emotion, aromatherapy can help reduce stress, alleviate anxiety, improve mood, enhance focus, and promote better sleep. Incorporating aromatherapy into daily practice provides a holistic way to support emotional resilience and overall health.

The accessibility and ease of use of essential oils make them an attractive option for those seeking natural methods to enhance their emotional well-being. However, it's important to use high-quality oils and follow safety guidelines to ensure the best results. Whether through diffusion, inhalation, or topical application, aromatherapy offers a valuable tool for improving emotional health and fostering a balanced, harmonious life. By embracing this ancient practice, individuals can tap into the profound healing power of nature to support their emotional and physical well-being.

Chapter 5: Essential Oils for Physical Health

- *Pain Relief and Inflammation*

- *Respiratory Health*

- *Digestive Health*

- *Skin Care and Healing*

- *Immune System Support*

Essential oils, with their potent natural compounds, have been cherished for centuries for their healing properties. These aromatic extracts from plants not only offer therapeutic benefits for emotional well-being but also play a significant role in supporting physical health. From alleviating pain and reducing inflammation to boosting respiratory and digestive health, essential oils are versatile tools in natural medicine. This chapter delves into how essential oils can enhance physical health, exploring their applications for pain relief, respiratory support, digestive health, skin care, and immune system support. By understanding the properties and benefits of these oils, you can harness their power to improve your overall well-being naturally and effectively.

Pain Relief and Inflammation

Essential oils have been used for centuries to alleviate pain and reduce inflammation. These natural remedies offer an alternative to conventional pain relief medications, providing both symptomatic relief and therapeutic benefits. Here's an in-depth look at how essential oils can be used for pain relief and inflammation:

1. Mechanisms of Action: Essential oils work through several mechanisms to reduce pain and inflammation. They contain bioactive compounds like terpenes, phenols, and esters, which have analgesic, anti-inflammatory, and antispasmodic properties. These compounds interact with the body's receptors and pathways to modulate pain perception and inflammatory responses.

2. Common Essential Oils for Pain Relief:

- **Lavender:** Known for its calming and analgesic properties, lavender oil can help relieve headaches, muscle pain, and joint discomfort. It also reduces anxiety, which can exacerbate pain.

- **Peppermint:** Peppermint oil contains menthol, which provides a cooling sensation and acts as a natural analgesic. It's effective for headaches, muscle aches, and joint pain.

- **Eucalyptus:** Eucalyptus oil has anti-inflammatory and analgesic effects. It's beneficial for conditions like arthritis, muscle soreness, and respiratory issues that cause discomfort.

- **Ginger:** Ginger oil is known for its warming and anti-inflammatory properties. It helps reduce pain associated with arthritis, muscle strains, and menstrual cramps.

- **Frankincense:** Frankincense oil has potent anti-inflammatory properties that can help with chronic pain conditions such as arthritis and inflammatory bowel disease.

3. Application Methods:

- **Topical Application:** Diluting essential oils with a carrier oil (like coconut or jojoba oil) and applying them to the affected area can provide targeted pain relief. Massage enhances absorption and increases circulation, further aiding in pain reduction.

- **Aromatherapy:** Inhaling essential oils through a

diffuser or inhaler can help manage pain, especially headaches and migraines. Aromatherapy also helps reduce stress and anxiety, which can indirectly alleviate pain.

- **Compresses:** Applying warm or cold compresses with added essential oils can be effective for localized pain relief. For example, a warm ginger compress can help with muscle pain, while a cold peppermint compress can reduce swelling and inflammation.

4. Scientific Evidence: Research supports the efficacy of essential oils for pain relief. Studies have shown that lavender oil reduces the intensity of migraine attacks and peppermint oil alleviates tension headaches. Eucalyptus oil has been found to decrease pain and improve joint mobility in arthritis patients.

In conclusion, essential oils offer a natural and effective way to manage pain and inflammation. By understanding their mechanisms, choosing the right oils, and applying them correctly, individuals can harness the therapeutic benefits of these potent natural remedies.

Respiratory Health

Essential oils are highly beneficial for respiratory health, providing relief from conditions like colds, flu, asthma, and allergies. Their antimicrobial, anti-inflammatory, and expectorant properties help clear airways, reduce inflammation, and fight infections. Here's a detailed exploration of how essential oils can support respiratory health:

1. Mechanisms of Action: Essential oils support respiratory health through several mechanisms. Their volatile compounds can kill or inhibit the growth of pathogens, reduce inflammation in the airways, and thin mucus, making it easier to expel. Additionally, their aromatic properties help soothe respiratory irritation and improve breathing.

2. Common Essential Oils for Respiratory Health:

- **Eucalyptus:** Eucalyptus oil is a powerful decongestant and expectorant. It helps clear mucus from the airways and sinuses, making it easier to breathe. Its antimicrobial properties also help fight respiratory infections.

- **Peppermint:** Peppermint oil contains menthol, which provides a cooling sensation and helps open up the nasal passages. It's effective for relieving congestion and improving airflow.

- **Tea Tree:** Tea tree oil has strong antimicrobial

properties that can help fight respiratory infections. It also reduces inflammation and soothes irritated airways.

- **Rosemary:** Rosemary oil acts as an expectorant, helping to expel mucus from the respiratory tract. It's also anti-inflammatory and can alleviate symptoms of asthma and bronchitis.

- **Lavender:** Lavender oil is calming and anti-inflammatory, making it beneficial for soothing respiratory irritation and promoting relaxation, which can improve breathing.

3. Application Methods:

- **Steam Inhalation:** Adding a few drops of essential oil to a bowl of hot water and inhaling the steam can provide immediate relief from congestion and respiratory discomfort. Eucalyptus and peppermint oils are particularly effective for this method.

- **Diffusion:** Using an essential oil diffuser to disperse oils into the air can help purify the air and provide ongoing respiratory support. This method is ideal for oils like tea tree and rosemary.

- **Chest Rubs:** Diluting essential oils with a carrier oil and applying them to the chest can help clear airways and reduce congestion. A peppermint or eucalyptus chest rub can be very effective.

- **Aromatherapy Inhalers:** Personal inhalers filled with essential oils can be used throughout the day for quick relief from respiratory symptoms.

4. Scientific Evidence: Numerous studies support the use of essential oils for respiratory health. Eucalyptus oil, for instance, has been shown to improve symptoms of chronic obstructive pulmonary disease (COPD) and asthma. Peppermint oil is effective in reducing symptoms of nasal congestion and sinusitis. Tea tree oil has demonstrated efficacy in fighting respiratory pathogens.

In conclusion, essential oils offer a natural and effective way to support respiratory health. By choosing the right oils and using them correctly, individuals can alleviate symptoms of respiratory conditions, improve breathing, and enhance overall respiratory wellness.

Digestive Health

Essential oils can play a significant role in supporting digestive health by alleviating symptoms such as indigestion, bloating, nausea, and stomach cramps. Their antispasmodic, anti-inflammatory, and carminative properties help regulate digestion and promote a healthy gastrointestinal system. Here's an in-depth look at how essential oils can benefit digestive health:

1. Mechanisms of Action: Essential oils support digestive health through various mechanisms. They can stimulate the production of digestive enzymes, relax the muscles of the gastrointestinal tract, reduce inflammation, and combat harmful bacteria. These actions help improve digestion, relieve discomfort, and promote overall gut health.

2. Common Essential Oils for Digestive Health:

- **Peppermint:** Peppermint oil is well-known for its ability to relieve digestive issues. It has antispasmodic properties that can reduce stomach cramps, bloating, and gas. It's also effective for alleviating symptoms of irritable bowel syndrome (IBS).

- **Ginger:** Ginger oil is a powerful digestive aid. It helps reduce nausea, improve digestion, and alleviate bloating and gas. It's particularly useful for motion sickness and morning sickness during pregnancy.

- **Fennel:** Fennel oil has carminative properties, meaning it helps reduce gas and bloating. It also stimulates digestion and can relieve constipation and indigestion.

- **Chamomile:** Chamomile oil is soothing and anti-inflammatory. It helps calm the digestive tract, reduce stomach cramps, and alleviate symptoms of indigestion and gastritis.

- **Lemon:** Lemon oil stimulates the production of digestive juices, improving digestion and reducing symptoms of indigestion. It also has detoxifying properties that support liver function.

3. Application Methods:

- **Topical Application:** Diluting essential oils with a carrier oil and massaging them onto the abdomen can provide relief from digestive discomfort. Peppermint and ginger oils are particularly effective for this method.

- **Inhalation:** Inhaling the aroma of essential oils can help reduce nausea and improve digestion. Using a diffuser or a personal inhaler with oils like ginger or lemon can be beneficial.

- **Internal Use (Caution):** Some essential oils can be taken internally to support digestion, but this should only be done under the guidance of a qualified healthcare provider. Oils like peppermint and ginger can be added to a carrier oil or diluted in water for ingestion.

4. Scientific Evidence: Research supports the use of essential oils for digestive health. Studies have shown that peppermint oil can significantly reduce symptoms of IBS, including abdominal pain and bloating. Ginger oil has been found to be effective in reducing nausea and improving overall digestive function. Fennel oil has been shown to relieve bloating and improve digestion in infants and adults.

In conclusion, essential oils offer a natural and effective way to support digestive health. By understanding their mechanisms, choosing the right oils, and applying them correctly, individuals can alleviate digestive discomfort, improve overall digestion, and promote a healthy gastrointestinal system.

Skin Care and Healing

Essential oils are powerful allies in skin care and healing, offering a range of benefits for maintaining healthy skin and addressing various skin concerns. Their antimicrobial, anti-inflammatory, and regenerative properties can treat conditions like acne, eczema, scars, and aging. Here's a detailed exploration of how essential oils can support skin health and healing:

1. Mechanisms of Action: Essential oils support skin health through several mechanisms. They can kill or inhibit the growth of pathogens that cause skin infections, reduce inflammation, promote wound healing, and stimulate the regeneration of skin cells. These actions help maintain healthy skin and accelerate the healing process.

2. Common Essential Oils for Skin Care and Healing:

- **Tea Tree:** Tea tree oil is renowned for its antimicrobial and anti-inflammatory properties. It's effective for treating acne, fungal infections, and minor cuts and scrapes.

- **Lavender:** Lavender oil is soothing and regenerative. It helps reduce inflammation, promote wound healing, and alleviate skin conditions like eczema and psoriasis.

- **Frankincense:** Frankincense oil has anti-inflammatory and skin-regenerative properties. It helps reduce the appearance of scars, wrinkles, and fine lines.

- **Chamomile:** Chamomile oil is calming and anti-inflammatory. It helps soothe irritated skin, reduce redness, and promote healing in conditions like dermatitis and eczema.

- **Rosehip:** Rosehip oil is rich in vitamins A and C, which promote skin regeneration and reduce the appearance of scars and hyperpigmentation.

3. Application Methods:

- **Topical Application:** Diluting essential oils with a carrier oil and applying them directly to the skin can provide targeted treatment for various skin concerns. For example, tea tree oil can be applied to acne spots, while lavender oil can be used on irritated skin.

- **Facial Steam:** Adding essential oils to a bowl of hot water and steaming the face can help open pores, cleanse the skin, and allow the oils to penetrate deeply. This method is beneficial for oils like tea tree and lavender.

- **Baths:** Adding essential oils to a warm bath can provide overall skin benefits. Oils like chamomile and lavender can soothe and moisturize the skin while promoting relaxation.

- **Compresses:** Applying warm or cold compresses with essential oils to the skin can provide relief from specific skin issues. For example, a cold chamomile compress can reduce inflammation and soothe irritated skin.

4. Scientific Evidence: Research supports the efficacy of essential oils for skin care and healing. Tea tree oil has been shown to be effective in treating acne and fungal infections. Lavender oil has demonstrated wound-healing properties and can reduce inflammation and scarring. Frankincense oil has been found to promote skin regeneration and reduce signs of aging.

In conclusion, essential oils offer a natural and effective way to support skin care and healing. By understanding their mechanisms, choosing the right oils, and applying them correctly, individuals can address various skin concerns, promote healthy skin, and accelerate the healing process.

Immune System Support

Essential oils can play a significant role in supporting the immune system by enhancing its ability to fight off infections and promoting overall health. Their antimicrobial, antiviral, and immune-stimulating properties help protect the body from pathogens and strengthen immune function. Here's an in-depth look at how essential oils can support the immune system:

1. Mechanisms of Action: Essential oils support the immune system through various mechanisms. They can kill or inhibit the growth of pathogens, reduce inflammation, and stimulate the production of immune cells. These actions help protect the body from infections and promote overall immune health.

2. Common Essential Oils for Immune System Support:

- **Tea Tree:** Tea tree oil is renowned for its antimicrobial properties. It's effective against a wide range of bacteria, viruses, and fungi, making it a valuable tool for immune support.

- **Eucalyptus:** Eucalyptus oil has antiviral and antibacterial properties. It helps clear respiratory infections and supports overall immune function.

- **Thyme:** Thyme oil is a powerful immune stimulant. It has strong antimicrobial properties and helps increase the production of white blood cells.

- **Oregano:** Oregano oil is highly antimicrobial and supports the immune system by fighting off infections. It's particularly effective against bacterial and viral pathogens.

- **Frankincense:** Frankincense oil has immunomodulatory properties. It helps regulate the immune system and reduce inflammation, promoting overall immune health.

3. Application Methods:

- **Diffusion:** Using an essential oil diffuser to disperse oils into the air can help purify the air and provide ongoing immune support. This method is ideal for oils like tea tree and eucalyptus.

- **Topical Application:** Diluting essential oils with a carrier oil and applying them to the skin can provide targeted immune support. For example, applying thyme or oregano oil to the soles of the feet can help boost immune function.

- **Steam Inhalation:** Adding essential oils to a bowl of hot water and inhaling the steam can provide immediate immune support, especially for respiratory infections. Eucalyptus and tea tree oils are particularly effective for this method.

- **Aromatherapy Inhalers:** Personal inhalers filled with essential oils can be used throughout the day for quick immune support.

4. Scientific Evidence: Research supports the use of essential oils for immune system support. Tea tree oil has been shown to be effective against a wide range of pathogens. Eucalyptus oil has demonstrated antiviral and antibacterial properties. Thyme and oregano oils have been found to stimulate immune function and fight off infections.

In conclusion, essential oils offer a natural and effective way to support the immune system. By understanding their mechanisms, choosing the right oils, and applying them correctly, individuals can enhance their immune function, protect their bodies from infections, and promote overall health and well-being. Incorporating essential oils into daily practice provides a holistic approach to maintaining a strong and resilient immune system.

Chapter 6: Essential Oils for Mental and Emotional Well-Being

- *Reducing Stress and Anxiety*

- *Enhancing Sleep Quality*

- *Boosting Mood and Energy*

- *Improving Concentration and Focus*

- *Managing Depression and Grief*

Essential oils have long been recognized for their profound impact on mental and emotional well-being. These potent plant extracts can help alleviate stress and anxiety, improve sleep quality, boost mood and energy, enhance concentration and focus, and assist in managing depression and grief. Yes, all of these benefits have already been discussed. By leveraging the therapeutic properties of essential oils, individuals can create a holistic approach to mental and emotional health. This chapter explores how essential oils can support various aspects of mental and emotional well-being.

Reducing Stress and Anxiety

Stress and anxiety are common issues in today's fast-paced world, affecting people's health and quality of life. Essential oils can be a powerful natural remedy to help manage these conditions by promoting relaxation and reducing tension.

1. Mechanisms of Action: Essential oils work to reduce stress and anxiety by influencing the limbic system, the part of the brain responsible for emotions and memory. When inhaled, the aromatic molecules of essential oils interact with the olfactory receptors, sending signals to the brain and triggering a calming response.

2. Common Essential Oils for Reducing Stress and Anxiety:

- **Lavender:** Lavender oil is well-known for its calming and relaxing properties. It helps reduce anxiety, improve mood, and promote a sense of calm.

- **Bergamot:** Bergamot oil has a unique ability to be both uplifting and calming. It can help reduce stress, improve mood, and alleviate anxiety.

- **Chamomile:** Chamomile oil is soothing and relaxing. It helps reduce stress and anxiety and promotes a sense of peace.

- **Frankincense:** Frankincense oil has grounding and calming properties. It helps reduce stress and anxiety and promotes mental clarity.

- **Ylang Ylang:** Ylang ylang oil has calming and anti-anxiety effects. It helps reduce stress, lower blood pressure, and promote relaxation.

3. Application Methods:

- **Diffusion:** Using an essential oil diffuser to disperse calming oils into the air can create a relaxing atmosphere and help reduce stress and anxiety throughout the day.

- **Inhalation:** Inhaling essential oils directly from the bottle or using an aromatherapy inhaler can provide immediate relief from stress and anxiety.

- **Topical Application:** Diluting essential oils with a carrier oil and applying them to pulse points (such as wrists, temples, and neck) can provide continuous stress relief.

- **Baths:** Adding a few drops of essential oils to a warm bath can create a relaxing experience and help reduce stress and anxiety.

4. Scientific Evidence: Numerous studies have demonstrated the effectiveness of essential oils in reducing stress and anxiety. Research has shown that inhaling lavender oil significantly reduces anxiety levels and improves mood. Bergamot oil has been found to reduce stress and improve psychological well-being. Chamomile oil has been shown to have anxiolytic effects and improve relaxation.

In conclusion, essential oils offer a natural and effective way to reduce stress and anxiety. By choosing the right oils and using them correctly, individuals can create a calming and relaxing environment, promote mental clarity, and improve overall emotional well-being.

Enhancing Sleep Quality

Quality sleep is essential for physical and mental health, yet many people struggle with sleep issues. Essential oils can help improve sleep quality by promoting relaxation, reducing insomnia, and creating a conducive environment for restful sleep.

1. Mechanisms of Action: Essential oils enhance sleep quality by calming the nervous system, reducing stress and anxiety, and promoting a sense of relaxation. The aromatic compounds in essential oils interact with the olfactory system, sending signals to the brain that induce relaxation and sleepiness.

2. Common Essential Oils for Enhancing Sleep Quality:

- **Lavender:** Lavender oil is one of the most popular essential oils for sleep. It helps reduce anxiety, promote relaxation, and improve overall sleep quality.

- **Chamomile:** Chamomile oil has soothing and calming properties that help promote relaxation and improve sleep.

- **Cedarwood:** Cedarwood oil has a sedative effect that helps promote relaxation and improve sleep quality.

- **Sandalwood:** Sandalwood oil has calming and grounding properties that help reduce anxiety and promote restful sleep.

- **Valerian:** Valerian oil is known for its sedative

properties. It helps reduce insomnia and improve sleep quality.

3. Application Methods:

- **Diffusion:** Using an essential oil diffuser in the bedroom can create a relaxing environment and promote restful sleep. Lavender, chamomile, and cedarwood oils are particularly effective for this method.

- **Topical Application:** Diluting essential oils with a carrier oil and applying them to the feet, wrists, or temples before bedtime can help promote relaxation and improve sleep quality.

- **Pillow Sprays:** Creating a pillow spray with essential oils can provide a calming scent that promotes sleep. Simply mix a few drops of essential oils with water in a spray bottle and mist onto your pillow before bed.

- **Baths:** Adding a few drops of essential oils to a warm bath before bedtime can help relax the body and mind, making it easier to fall asleep.

4. Scientific Evidence: Research supports the use of essential oils for improving sleep quality. Studies have shown that inhaling lavender oil significantly improves sleep quality and reduces insomnia. Chamomile oil has

been found to have a calming effect that promotes relaxation and improves sleep. Valerian oil has been shown to reduce the time it takes to fall asleep and improve overall sleep quality.

In conclusion, essential oils offer a natural and effective way to enhance sleep quality. By choosing the right oils and using them correctly, individuals can create a relaxing bedtime routine, reduce insomnia, and improve overall sleep quality.

Boosting Mood and Energy

Essential oils can be powerful tools for boosting mood and energy levels. Their uplifting and invigorating properties help improve mental clarity, increase energy, and enhance overall emotional well-being.

1. Mechanisms of Action: Essential oils boost mood and energy by stimulating the brain and nervous system. The aromatic compounds in essential oils interact with the olfactory system, sending signals to the brain that promote alertness, improve mood, and increase energy levels.

2. Common Essential Oils for Boosting Mood and Energy:

- **Citrus Oils (Lemon, Orange, Grapefruit):** Citrus oils are known for their uplifting and invigorating properties. They help improve mood, increase energy, and reduce fatigue.

- **Peppermint:** Peppermint oil has stimulating properties that help increase alertness, improve mental clarity, and boost energy levels.

- **Rosemary:** Rosemary oil is known for its ability to improve cognitive function, increase energy, and reduce mental fatigue.

- **Bergamot:** Bergamot oil has a unique ability to be both uplifting and calming. It helps improve mood, reduce stress, and increase energy.

- **Eucalyptus:** Eucalyptus oil has invigorating properties that help improve mental clarity, increase energy, and reduce fatigue.

3. Application Methods:

- **Diffusion:** Using an essential oil diffuser to disperse uplifting oils into the air can create an energizing environment and help improve mood and energy levels throughout the day.

- **Inhalation:** Inhaling essential oils directly from the bottle or using an aromatherapy inhaler can provide immediate relief from fatigue and improve mood and energy.

- **Topical Application:** Diluting essential oils with a carrier oil and applying them to pulse points (such as wrists, temples, and neck) can provide continuous mood and energy support.

- **Sprays:** Creating a room spray with essential oils can provide an invigorating scent that boosts mood and energy. Simply mix a few drops of essential oils with water in a spray bottle and mist around the room.

4. Scientific Evidence: Research supports the use of essential oils for boosting mood and energy levels. Studies have shown that inhaling citrus oils significantly improves mood and reduces fatigue. Peppermint oil has been found to increase alertness and improve cognitive performance. Rosemary oil has demonstrated efficacy in improving cognitive function and reducing mental fatigue.

5. Precautions and Safety: While essential oils are generally safe when used properly, it is important to use them with caution. Always dilute essential oils before applying them to the skin to avoid irritation or sensitization. Conduct a patch test to check for allergies.

Pregnant women, nursing mothers, and individuals with specific health conditions should consult a healthcare provider before using essential oils.

In conclusion, essential oils offer a natural and effective way to boost mood and energy levels. By choosing the right oils and using them correctly, individuals can create an uplifting and invigorating environment, improve mental clarity, and enhance overall emotional well-being.

Improving Concentration and Focus

Essential oils can be valuable tools for improving concentration and focus. Their stimulating and clarifying properties help enhance cognitive function, increase attention span, and reduce mental fatigue.

1. Mechanisms of Action: Essential oils improve concentration and focus by stimulating the brain and nervous system. The aromatic compounds in essential oils interact with the olfactory system, sending signals to the brain that promote alertness, enhance cognitive function, and improve mental clarity.

2. Common Essential Oils for Improving Concentration and Focus:

- **Peppermint:** Peppermint oil is known for its stimulating properties. It helps increase alertness, improve mental clarity, and enhance cognitive function, making it easier to concentrate and maintain focus.

- **Rosemary:** Rosemary oil has cognitive-enhancing properties that help improve memory, concentration, and mental clarity.

- **Lemon:** Lemon oil is uplifting and invigorating. It helps improve focus, increase alertness, and enhance cognitive performance.

- **Basil:** Basil oil has a clarifying effect that helps improve mental clarity, increase focus, and reduce mental fatigue.

- **Frankincense:** Frankincense oil has grounding and calming properties that help improve focus, enhance concentration, and promote mental clarity.

3. Application Methods:

- **Diffusion:** Using an essential oil diffuser to disperse focusing oils into the air can create a conducive environment for concentration and focus. Oils like peppermint, rosemary, and lemon are particularly effective for this method.

- **Topical Application:** Diluting essential oils with a carrier oil and applying them to pulse points (such as wrists, temples, and neck) can provide continuous support for concentration and focus throughout the day.

- **Aromatherapy Inhalers:** Personal inhalers filled with essential oils can be used as needed throughout the day to enhance mental clarity and improve focus.

- **Study Blends:** Creating a study blend by combining oils like rosemary, peppermint, and lemon can enhance cognitive function and support concentration during study or work sessions.

4. Scientific Evidence: Research supports the use of essential oils for improving concentration and focus. Studies have shown that inhaling peppermint oil can enhance memory and cognitive performance. Rosemary oil has been found to improve cognitive function and increase alertness. Lemon oil has demonstrated efficacy in improving mood, reducing stress, and enhancing cognitive performance.

In conclusion, essential oils offer a natural and effective way to improve concentration and focus. By choosing the right oils and using them correctly, individuals can enhance cognitive function, increase mental clarity, and maintain focus during tasks and activities.

Managing Depression and Grief

Essential oils can be supportive in managing depression and grief by promoting emotional balance, providing comfort, and uplifting mood. While not a replacement for professional treatment, they can complement therapeutic approaches and offer additional emotional support.

1. Mechanisms of Action: Essential oils can help manage depression and grief by affecting the limbic system and influencing emotions. Their aromatic compounds can stimulate the release of neurotransmitters like serotonin and dopamine, which are involved in regulating mood and emotions.

2. Common Essential Oils for Managing Depression and Grief:

- **Bergamot:** Bergamot oil has uplifting and calming properties that can help alleviate symptoms of depression and anxiety. It promotes relaxation and reduces stress.

- **Ylang Ylang:** Ylang ylang oil is soothing and uplifting. It helps reduce feelings of sadness and promotes emotional well-being.

- **Geranium:** Geranium oil has balancing properties that

can help stabilize emotions, reduce anxiety, and uplift mood.

- **Clary Sage:** Clary sage oil has antidepressant and mood-enhancing properties. It helps reduce stress and promote relaxation.

- **Lavender:** Lavender oil is calming and relaxing, making it beneficial for reducing anxiety and promoting emotional balance.

3. Application Methods:

- **Diffusion:** Using an essential oil diffuser to disperse uplifting oils into the air can create a comforting atmosphere and support emotional well-being. Oils like bergamot, ylang ylang, and geranium are particularly effective for this method.

- **Topical Application:** Diluting essential oils with a carrier oil and applying them to pulse points (such as wrists, temples, and neck) can provide continuous emotional support throughout the day.

- **Baths:** Adding a few drops of essential oils to a warm bath can create a calming and soothing experience that promotes relaxation and emotional balance.

- **Massage:** Incorporating essential oils into massage therapy can help alleviate tension, reduce stress, and promote emotional well-being.

4. Scientific Evidence: Research on essential oils for managing depression and grief is ongoing. While preliminary studies show promising results, more research is needed to fully understand their efficacy. Some studies have demonstrated that inhaling bergamot oil can reduce stress and improve mood. Lavender oil has been shown to have anxiolytic and mood-stabilizing effects.

In conclusion, essential oils offer a supportive and holistic approach to managing depression and grief. By choosing the right oils and integrating them into daily self-care routines, individuals can enhance emotional well-being, find comfort during difficult times, and support overall mental health.

This chapter demonstrates the diverse ways in which essential oils can be used to support mental and emotional well-being. Whether reducing stress and anxiety, enhancing sleep quality, boosting mood and energy, improving concentration and focus, or managing depression and grief, essential oils offer a natural and effective tool for promoting overall emotional health. Integrating these oils into daily routines can provide therapeutic benefits and contribute to a balanced and resilient mind.

Chapter 7: Integrating Essential Oils into Daily Life

- *Essential Oils in Personal Care Products*

- *Household Cleaning with Essential Oils*

- *Cooking and Food Preservation*

- *Pet Care and Safety*

- *Travel Tips with Essential Oils*

Essential oils are versatile and can be integrated into various aspects of daily life beyond aromatherapy. From personal care products to household cleaning, cooking, pet care, and travel, essential oils offer natural alternatives with therapeutic benefits. This chapter explores practical ways to incorporate essential oils into daily routines.

Essential Oils in Personal Care Products

Essential oils can enhance personal care products, offering natural fragrance and therapeutic benefits for skin and hair.

1. Skincare: Essential oils like lavender, tea tree, and frankincense are commonly used in skincare products for their antibacterial, anti-inflammatory, and rejuvenating properties. They can be added to moisturizers, serums, and facial masks to promote healthy skin.

2. Hair Care: Oils such as rosemary, peppermint, and cedarwood are beneficial for hair care. They stimulate the scalp, promote hair growth, and add shine when infused into shampoos, conditioners, and hair oils.

3. Body Care: Citrus oils like lemon and grapefruit are refreshing additions to body scrubs and lotions, offering a natural fragrance and uplifting mood.

4. DIY Recipes: Creating DIY personal care products allows customization. For example, mixing lavender and chamomile oils with coconut oil makes a soothing body lotion ideal for bedtime relaxation.

Household Cleaning with Essential Oils

Essential oils provide effective alternatives to commercial cleaning products, offering natural antimicrobial and antiseptic properties.

1. All-Purpose Cleaner: Create a DIY cleaner by combining vinegar, water, and tea tree oil. This mixture effectively cleans surfaces and kills bacteria.

2. Air Fresheners: Diffuse oils like lemon, eucalyptus, and peppermint to purify the air and provide a fresh scent without synthetic chemicals.

3. Laundry: Add a few drops of lavender or eucalyptus oil to laundry detergent for natural fragrance and antimicrobial benefits.

4. Disinfectant Spray: Mix water, vodka, and lavender oil in a spray bottle for a homemade disinfectant that is safe and pleasant-smelling.

Cooking and Food Preservation

Essential oils can be used in cooking and food preservation to enhance flavor and provide health benefits.

1. Flavor Enhancers: Oils like basil, oregano, and lemon add depth to dishes without the need for fresh herbs. Remember, a little goes a long way.

2. Food Preservation: Use oils with antimicrobial properties, such as thyme or cinnamon, when preserving foods like jams or pickles to inhibit bacterial growth naturally.

3. Baking: Incorporate oils like orange or peppermint into baking recipes for unique flavors in cakes, cookies, or chocolates.

4. Beverages: Add a drop of peppermint oil to hot chocolate or lemon oil to tea for a refreshing twist.

Pet Care and Safety

When used correctly, essential oils can benefit pets, but caution is essential due to their sensitive nature.

1. Aromatherapy: Use calming oils like lavender or chamomile in a diffuser to soothe anxious pets.

2. DIY Pet Shampoo: Create a gentle shampoo with diluted lavender or cedarwood oil to cleanse and deodorize fur naturally.

3. Tick and Flea Prevention: Use oils like citronella or geranium in a spray diluted with water to repel insects from pet bedding.

4. Safety: Consult a veterinarian before using essential oils around pets, especially cats and smaller animals, as some oils can be toxic to them.

Travel Tips with Essential Oils

Essential oils are compact and versatile travel companions, providing comfort and support on the go.

1. Stress Relief: Carry a rollerball blend of lavender and bergamot for calming effects during travel.

2. Immune Support: Inhale eucalyptus or tea tree oil from a handkerchief to maintain respiratory health in crowded areas.

3. Motion Sickness: Ginger or peppermint oil applied to the wrists or inhaled can alleviate nausea during travel.

4. First Aid: Pack a small kit with lavender oil for minor cuts or insect bites.

Integrating essential oils into daily life enhances well-being naturally. Whether enhancing personal care, cleaning, cooking, caring for pets, or traveling, these oils offer multifaceted benefits and contribute to a healthier lifestyle.

Chapter 8: Essential Oils for Specific Populations

- *Essential Oils for Children*

- *Essential Oils for the Elderly*

- *Essential Oils for Pregnant and Nursing Women*

- *Essential Oils for Athletes*

- *Essential Oils for Men*

Essential oils offer tailored benefits and considerations for specific populations, including children, the elderly, pregnant and nursing women, athletes, and men. Each group requires a nuanced approach to ensure safe and effective use of these natural remedies.

Essential Oils for Children

Essential oils can be beneficial for children when used appropriately and with caution. They offer gentle support for common childhood concerns such as sleep issues, skin irritations, and emotional well-being. Lavender oil, known for its calming properties, can help children relax before bedtime and promote better sleep quality. Chamomile oil, with its soothing effects, is often used to alleviate minor skin irritations or discomfort.

Safety is crucial when using essential oils with children due to their sensitive skin and developing respiratory systems. Oils should always be diluted properly before application. It's recommended to use a lower dilution ratio for younger children and to avoid oils that may be too strong or cause adverse reactions.

Practical applications include diffusing oils in their bedroom to create a calming environment, applying diluted oils topically for gentle massages, or using them in inhalation blends for emotional support. These methods not only address specific concerns but also contribute to a nurturing and healthy atmosphere for children's well-being.

Essential Oils for the Elderly

Essential oils can play a significant role in supporting the health and well-being of elderly individuals. They offer natural remedies for various age-related issues such as joint discomfort, sleep disturbances, and emotional stress. Lavender oil, revered for its calming effects, can help reduce anxiety and improve sleep quality in older adults. Frankincense oil, known for its grounding properties, is beneficial for promoting emotional balance and supporting overall mental well-being.

When using essential oils with the elderly, it's essential to consider their individual health conditions and sensitivities. Elderly individuals often have more delicate skin and may be taking medications that could interact with essential oils. Therefore, oils should be diluted appropriately and patch tested before widespread use.

Practical applications include using diluted oils in massage oils or creams for soothing massages that can alleviate muscle tension and promote relaxation. Diffusing oils in living spaces can also provide emotional support and create a comforting atmosphere, contributing to overall well-being and quality of life.

Essential Oils for Pregnant and Nursing Women

Pregnant and nursing women can benefit from the therapeutic properties of essential oils to support their physical and emotional health. Oils such as lavender are popular for their calming effects, helping to reduce stress and promote relaxation during pregnancy. Ginger oil is often used to alleviate nausea associated with morning sickness, while citrus oils like lemon can provide mood enhancement and a refreshing aroma.

Safety is paramount when using essential oils during pregnancy and breastfeeding. It's crucial to consult with a healthcare provider to ensure that chosen oils are safe and appropriate for individual circumstances. Oils should be highly diluted (1% or less) for topical application to minimize absorption and potential effects on the developing fetus or breastfeeding infant.

Practical applications include using essential oils in aromatherapy through diffusion or diluted in carrier oils for gentle massage. These methods can provide emotional support, alleviate minor discomforts, and enhance overall well-being during this special time of life.

Essential Oils for Athletes

Athletes can benefit greatly from incorporating essential oils into their training and recovery routines. Essential oils offer natural solutions to enhance performance, aid in recovery, and support overall wellness during intense physical activities. Peppermint oil, known for its invigorating properties, can help boost energy levels and improve focus before workouts. Eucalyptus oil is valued for its respiratory benefits, aiding in clear breathing and supporting respiratory health during exercise.

Safety considerations are crucial for athletes, given their active lifestyles and potential for skin sensitivities. Oils should be properly diluted and tested for individual tolerance before regular use.

Practical applications include using pre-workout blends to enhance mental focus and energy, applying post-workout massages with soothing oils to aid in muscle recovery, and using inhalation blends to support respiratory function. These applications can help athletes optimize performance, recover effectively, and maintain overall well-being throughout their training regimens.

Essential Oils for Men

Men can integrate essential oils into their daily routines to support various aspects of health, from skincare and grooming to emotional well-being and vitality. Essential oils offer natural solutions for maintaining healthy skin, promoting relaxation, and enhancing overall wellness. Tea tree oil, known for its antibacterial properties, is often used in skincare products to help manage acne and maintain clear skin. Cedarwood oil, with its grounding and calming effects, can promote emotional balance and relaxation after a long day.

Practical applications include incorporating essential oils into daily hygiene routines, such as using them in aftershaves, moisturizers, or beard oils. Diffusing oils in living spaces can provide emotional support and create a pleasant atmosphere, while topical application with carrier oils can support skin health and overall well-being.

Essential oils offer men a natural and versatile approach to enhancing health, supporting emotional well-being, and maintaining vitality in daily life. By selecting oils that align with personal preferences and needs, men can integrate these aromatic treasures into their routines for holistic wellness benefits.

Chapter 9: Advanced Applications and Blending Techniques

- *Understanding Notes and Blending Ratios*

- *Creating Therapeutic Blends*

- *Crafting Perfumes and Fragrances*

- *Making Balms and Salves*

- *Troubleshooting Common Blending Issues*

Essential oils offer a vast array of applications beyond basic use, allowing enthusiasts to delve into advanced techniques such as understanding notes and blending ratios, creating therapeutic blends, crafting perfumes and fragrances, making balms and salves, and troubleshooting common blending issues. Each of these techniques requires a blend of artistry, scientific understanding, and practical application to harness the full potential of essential oils. We've already touched on all of this, but now we will dive deeper in.

Understanding Notes and Blending Ratios

In the world of perfumery and aromatherapy, understanding notes is crucial to creating harmonious and balanced blends. Notes refer to the different stages of scent perception in a fragrance, categorized as top, middle (heart), and base notes. Each note contributes to the overall scent profile and longevity of a blend.

Blending ratios determine the proportion of each note in a blend. For example, a balanced blend might consist of 30% top notes, 50% middle notes, and 20% base notes. However, these ratios can vary depending on the desired fragrance profile and intended therapeutic effects.

In perfumery and aromatherapy, notes refer to the different stages of scent perception within a fragrance. These notes are categorized into three main categories:

1. Top Notes:

- These are the initial scents perceived upon application and are typically light, fresh, and volatile.

- Examples include citrus oils like bergamot, lemongrass, or floral notes like neroli.

- Top notes provide the first impression of a fragrance and are often uplifting and invigorating.

2. Middle (Heart) Notes:

- Middle notes emerge once the top notes have dissipated and form the main body of the fragrance.

- They are fuller and more rounded in scent, contributing to the overall character and complexity of the blend.

- Examples include floral oils like lavender, geranium, or herbal notes like rosemary.

- Middle notes provide depth and balance to the fragrance, influencing its overall theme.

3. Base Notes:

- Base notes are the foundation of the blend, offering depth, richness, and longevity to the fragrance.

- They emerge once the middle notes have evaporated and provide a lingering scent that lasts.

- Examples include woody oils like cedarwood, sandalwood, or resinous notes like frankincense.

- Base notes often have grounding and stabilizing effects, anchoring the fragrance and enhancing its lasting power.

Understanding these notes allows perfumers and aromatherapists to create harmonious blends that evolve over time, providing a rich sensory experience. By strategically combining oils from each note category, practitioners can achieve a well-rounded fragrance profile that resonates with the desired emotional or therapeutic effect.

Importance of Blending Ratios

Blending ratios determine the proportion of each note within a blend, influencing its overall balance, intensity, and effectiveness. While there are no strict rules, understanding how to balance these ratios is essential for creating blends that achieve specific outcomes.

1. Achieving Balance:

- Proper blending ratios ensure that no single note dominates the blend excessively, creating a harmonious synergy among the oils.

- For example, a balanced blend might consist of 30% top notes, 50% middle notes, and 20% base notes, although ratios can vary based on the desired fragrance profile and therapeutic goals.

2. Enhancing Therapeutic Benefits:

- Each note category offers unique therapeutic properties that can be enhanced through proper blending ratios.

- For instance, blending calming top notes like lavender with grounding base notes like sandalwood can create a blend that promotes relaxation and emotional balance.

3. Ensuring Longevity:

- Base notes, with their lower volatility, contribute to the longevity of the fragrance, ensuring that the blend remains aromatic for an extended period.

- By understanding and utilizing base notes effectively, practitioners can create blends with lasting aromatic effects, suitable for applications such as perfumery or long-term aromatherapy benefits.

Practical Application

In practice, understanding notes and blending ratios involves experimentation, creativity, and a deep knowledge of each oil's properties. Perfumers and aromatherapists often keep detailed records of their blends, noting the effects of different ratios on scent profile and therapeutic outcomes. They may also conduct sensory evaluations to assess how blends evolve over time and under different conditions.

Mastering the art of understanding notes and blending ratios allows practitioners to create personalized fragrances, therapeutic blends, and effective remedies tailored to individual preferences and needs. It empowers them to harness the full potential of essential oils, offering diverse sensory experiences and enhancing well-being through the power of scent.

Creating Therapeutic Blends

Creating therapeutic blends with essential oils involves combining oils strategically to achieve specific health or emotional benefits. This process requires knowledge of each oil's properties, synergistic effects, and therapeutic applications. Here's a deeper exploration into the art and science of crafting therapeutic blends:

To create a therapeutic blend, start with a clear intention and understanding of the desired outcome. Consider the individual properties of each oil and how they synergize together. Experimentation and testing are crucial to finding the right balance and potency for the desired effect.

Understanding Therapeutic Blends

Therapeutic blends aim to harness the natural healing properties of essential oils to address specific concerns such as stress relief, immune support, pain management, and emotional balance. Each essential oil carries unique chemical constituents that contribute to its therapeutic effects, making careful selection and blending essential.

1. Selecting Oils Based on Properties:

- **Calming and Relaxing:** Oils like lavender, chamomile, and bergamot are renowned for their calming effects, reducing anxiety and promoting relaxation.

- **Energizing and Uplifting:** Citrus oils such as lemon, orange, and grapefruit are known for their uplifting properties, boosting mood and energy levels.

- **Anti-inflammatory:** Oils like peppermint, eucalyptus, and tea tree possess anti-inflammatory properties, beneficial for easing muscle tension and joint discomfort.

- **Antimicrobial:** Tea tree, eucalyptus, and thyme oils are effective against bacteria and viruses, supporting immune function.

- **Balancing Hormones:** Clary sage, geranium, and ylang-ylang oils can help regulate hormonal balance and alleviate menstrual discomfort.

2. Synergistic Blending:

- Combining oils with complementary properties can enhance their overall effectiveness. For example, blending calming oils like lavender and chamomile with grounding oils like frankincense can create a blend that promotes relaxation and emotional stability.

- Consider the aromatic profile, intensity, and potential interactions of each oil when creating blends. Experimentation and small batch testing are essential to finding the right balance and potency.

3. Creating Balanced Formulations:

- Start with a clear intention for the therapeutic blend, whether it's to alleviate a specific symptom, enhance emotional well-being, or support overall health.

- Use a carrier oil such as jojoba, sweet almond, or coconut oil to dilute the essential oils and ensure safe application. The typical dilution ratio for therapeutic blends is 1-3%, depending on the intended use and sensitivity of the skin.

- Keep notes of each blend's ingredients, ratios, and effects for future reference and adjustment.

Practical Application

1. Stress Relief Blend:

- **Ingredients:** Lavender, bergamot, and frankincense essential oils.

- **Purpose:** Promotes relaxation, reduces stress and anxiety.

- **Blend Ratio:** 2 drops lavender, 2 drops bergamot, 1 drop frankincense per 10ml of carrier oil.

- **Application:** Massage onto pulse points or diffuse in the air during times of stress.

2. Immune Support Blend:

- **Ingredients:** Tea tree, eucalyptus, and lemon essential oils.

- **Purpose:** Supports immune function, clears respiratory passages.

- **Blend Ratio:** 2 drops tea tree, 2 drops eucalyptus, 1 drop lemon per 10ml of carrier oil.

- **Application:** Apply to chest and throat area or use in a steam inhalation.

3. Muscle Relief Blend:

- **Ingredients:** Peppermint, lavender, and marjoram essential oils.

- **Purpose:** Eases muscle tension, promotes relaxation.

- **Blend Ratio:** 2 drops peppermint, 3 drops lavender, 1 drop marjoram per 10ml of carrier oil.

- **Application:** Massage onto sore muscles or add to a warm bath.

Creating therapeutic blends with essential oils involves a blend of science, creativity, and sensitivity to individual needs. By understanding the properties of each oil and how they interact, practitioners can formulate blends that promote physical healing, emotional balance, and overall well-being. Experimentation and personalized adjustments are key to discovering effective blends that resonate with specific health goals and preferences.

Crafting Perfumes and Fragrances

Creating perfumes and fragrances with essential oils is a fascinating blend of artistry, science, and sensory exploration. Unlike commercial perfumes that often rely on synthetic ingredients, natural perfumes made with essential oils offer a unique olfactory experience while potentially providing therapeutic benefits. Here's a detailed look into the process of crafting perfumes and fragrances:

Creating perfumes involves selecting complementary oils based on their aromatic profiles and blending them to achieve a desired fragrance. This process requires patience and experimentation to achieve a balanced and appealing scent. Perfume-making also involves considerations such as the longevity of the scent (affected by the notes used), the concentration of oils, and the carrier medium (e.g., alcohol, carrier oils).

Understanding Perfume Creation

Perfume-making involves selecting and combining essential oils to achieve a desired scent profile that resonates with personal preferences or specific purposes. Each essential oil contributes its unique aroma, intensity, and longevity to the blend, creating a complex and multi-layered fragrance.

1. Selection of Essential Oils:

- **Top Notes:** These are the initial scents perceived upon application, often light, fresh, and uplifting. Examples include citrus oils like bergamot, lemon, or floral notes like neroli.

- **Middle Notes (Heart Notes):** These notes emerge once the top notes have dissipated and form the main body of the fragrance. They are fuller and more rounded in scent, providing depth and character. Examples include floral oils like rose, lavender, or spicy notes like cinnamon.

- **Base Notes:** Base notes are the foundation of the blend, offering depth, richness, and longevity to the fragrance. They emerge once the middle notes have evaporated and provide a lingering scent that lasts. Examples include woody oils like cedarwood, sandalwood, or resinous notes like frankincense.

2. Blending Techniques:

- **Understanding Ratios:** Blending ratios determine the proportion of each note in the perfume, influencing its overall balance and character. A typical ratio might be 30% top notes, 50% middle notes, and 20% base notes, though this can vary based on desired fragrance intensity and longevity.

- **Layering:** Layering involves adding oils in sequential stages, starting with base notes, followed by middle notes, and finishing with top notes. This technique allows each layer to harmonize and evolve over time, creating a dynamic fragrance experience.

3. Dilution and Carrier Medium:

- Essential oils are highly concentrated and must be diluted before application to the skin. Carrier oils like jojoba, sweet almond, or fractionated coconut oil are commonly used to dilute essential oils in perfumery.

- Alcohol-based perfumes involve diluting essential oils in high-proof ethanol or vodka, allowing for quick evaporation and long-lasting fragrance.

Crafting a Natural Perfume

1. Scent Profile and Intention:

- Begin with a clear intention for the perfume, whether it's to create a calming blend for relaxation, an uplifting blend for energy, or a complex fragrance reminiscent of a specific memory or place.

- Experiment with different combinations of essential oils to achieve the desired scent profile, considering how each oil contributes to the overall aroma and emotional response.

2. Testing and Refining:

- Start with small batches to test different blends and ratios. Keep detailed notes of each formulation, including ingredients, ratios, and the sensory experience.

- Allow the perfume to mature over time, as the scent may evolve and mellow with aging. Test the fragrance on your skin to assess its longevity and how it interacts with your body chemistry.

3. Personalization and Creativity:

- Perfume-making is a highly personal and creative process. Experiment with unconventional pairings, explore new scent combinations, and trust your intuition to create unique and memorable fragrances.

- Consider seasonal influences and occasions when crafting perfumes. Lighter, floral scents may be preferred for spring and summer, while richer, spicier blends can evoke warmth in autumn and winter.

Ethical and Sustainable Practices

1. Sourcing: Choose high-quality, sustainably sourced essential oils to ensure purity and ethical practices in perfume-making.

- Consider the environmental impact of sourcing practices and opt for suppliers committed to fair trade and sustainable harvesting methods.

2. Storage: Store perfumes in dark, glass bottles away from heat and light to preserve their potency and fragrance integrity.

- Label each perfume bottle with the ingredients and date of creation for future reference and adjustments.

Crafting perfumes and fragrances with essential oils is an enriching journey that combines artistic expression with therapeutic potential. By understanding the properties of each oil, experimenting with blending techniques, and embracing creativity, perfumers can create personalized scents that not only delight the senses but also contribute to overall well-being. Whether for personal use or as a thoughtful gift, natural perfumes made with essential oils offer a sustainable and aromatic alternative to commercial fragrances, enhancing daily rituals and uplifting the spirit through the power of scent.

Making Balms and Salves

Balms and salves are practical applications of essential oils for topical use, offering benefits such as skin nourishment, wound healing, and pain relief. Balms typically contain a base of beeswax or another solid oil, melted together with carrier oils and essential oils. Here's a detailed exploration of how to create these beneficial formulations:

Understanding Balms and Salves

1. Benefits and Uses:

- **Skin Nourishment:** Balms and salves provide hydration and nutrients to the skin, promoting overall skin health and elasticity.

- **Wound Healing:** Certain essential oils like lavender, tea tree, and helichrysum possess antiseptic and healing properties, beneficial for minor cuts, scrapes, and insect bites.

- **Pain Relief:** Balms infused with essential oils such as peppermint, eucalyptus, and ginger can provide relief from muscle soreness, joint pain, and headaches when applied topically.

2. Basic Ingredients:

- **Carrier Oils:** Commonly used carrier oils include coconut oil, shea butter, cocoa butter, almond oil, or olive oil. These oils serve as a base, providing nourishment and aiding in the absorption of essential oils into the skin.

- **Beeswax or Alternative Solidifier:** Beeswax is often used to solidify balms and salves while providing a protective barrier on the skin. Alternatives like candelilla wax or soy wax can be used for vegan formulations.

- **Essential Oils:** Select essential oils based on their therapeutic properties and intended use. Examples include lavender for calming and soothing effects, peppermint for cooling relief, and chamomile for anti-inflammatory benefits.

Creating Balms and Salves

To make a balm or salve, start by melting the base ingredients and then incorporating essential oils known for their therapeutic properties. For example, a soothing muscle balm might include peppermint and eucalyptus oils for cooling and pain relief, blended with a moisturizing base like shea butter or coconut oil.

1. Recipe Formulation:

- **Basic Ratio:** A typical ratio for balms is approximately 1 part beeswax (or alternative solidifier) to 4-5 parts carrier oil. This ratio can be adjusted depending on the desired consistency and intended use.

- **Melting and Mixing:** Melt the beeswax and carrier oils together using a double boiler or microwave. Once melted, remove from heat and stir in essential oils. Stir thoroughly to ensure even distribution.

- **Cooling and Setting:** Pour the mixture into clean, sterilized containers such as glass jars or tins. Allow the balm to cool and solidify at room temperature. Avoid placing hot balms in the refrigerator, as rapid cooling may affect texture and consistency.

2. Customizing for Specific Needs:

- **Muscle Relief Balm:** Combine coconut oil, beeswax, and essential oils such as peppermint, eucalyptus, and lavender for a soothing balm to relieve sore muscles and joints.

- **Skin Healing Salve:** Use shea butter, calendula-infused oil, beeswax, and essential oils like tea tree and lavender to create a healing salve for minor cuts, burns, or dry skin patches.

- **Lip Balm:** Mix beeswax, cocoa butter, coconut oil, and a hint of peppermint essential oil for a nourishing lip balm that moisturizes and protects lips.

3. Application and Storage:

- Apply balms and salves directly to clean, dry skin as needed. Massage gently until absorbed.

- Store balms in a cool, dry place away from direct sunlight to preserve their potency and consistency. Use within 6-12 months, as natural formulations may oxidize over time.

Safety Considerations

1. **Patch Testing:** Before widespread use, perform a patch test on a small area of skin to check for any allergic reactions or sensitivities to the ingredients.

- **Consultation:** Seek advice from a qualified aromatherapist or healthcare professional, especially if pregnant, nursing, or using essential oils on children.

Creating balms and salves with essential oils offers a natural and effective way to support skin health, promote healing, and provide targeted relief from discomfort. Whether for personal use or as thoughtful gifts, these formulations can be customized with various essential oils and carrier oils to address specific needs and preferences. By mastering the art of balm and salve making, individuals can enjoy the benefits of aromatherapy in everyday skincare routines, fostering wellness through the power of botanicals and essential oils.

Troubleshooting Common Blending Issues

Even seasoned practitioners encounter challenges when blending essential oils. Common issues include overpowering scents, lack of synergy among oils, or unexpected reactions on the skin. Troubleshooting requires careful observation, adjusting ratios, and sometimes starting over with a fresh approach.

To troubleshoot blending issues, consider the following tips:

- Start with small batches to minimize waste if adjustments are needed.

- Keep detailed notes of each blend's ingredients and ratios for future reference.

- Experiment with different combinations and observe how oils interact over time.

- Seek advice from experienced aromatherapists or perfumers for guidance on complex blends or persistent issues.

Mastering advanced applications and blending techniques with essential oils requires patience, creativity, and a willingness to learn from both successes and challenges. Whether crafting therapeutic blends, designing personalized fragrances, or formulating practical balms, the journey of exploration and discovery in aromatherapy offers endless possibilities for enhancing well-being and enjoyment through the power of scent.

Chapter 10: Building Your Essential Oil Toolkit

- *Must-Have Essential Oils for Beginners*

- *Essential Oil Storage and Shelf Life*

- *Tools and Accessories for Essential Oil Use*

- *Continuing Education and Certification*

- *Resources and Communities for Essential Oil Enthusiasts*

Embarking on a journey with essential oils involves assembling a toolkit that includes a selection of oils, proper storage solutions, essential tools and accessories, opportunities for education and certification, and a supportive community. Here's a comprehensive guide to building your essential oil toolkit:

Must-Have Essential Oils for Beginners

For beginners, selecting essential oils that offer versatility and a range of therapeutic benefits is key. Here are some must-have essential oils to start your collection:

1. Lavender: Known for its calming and soothing properties, lavender is a versatile oil that promotes relaxation and supports skin health.

2. Peppermint: Invigorating and refreshing, peppermint essential oil helps alleviate headaches, supports digestion, and provides a cooling sensation for muscle relief.

3. Tea Tree: With powerful antimicrobial properties, tea tree oil is effective for treating acne, minor cuts, and fungal infections while supporting overall skin health.

4. Lemon: Bright and uplifting, lemon oil is renowned for its cleansing properties and can be used to purify the air, uplift mood, and support immune function.

5. Eucalyptus: Ideal for respiratory support, eucalyptus oil helps clear nasal congestion, soothes muscles, and promotes relaxation during cold and flu season.

6. Frankincense: Revered for its grounding and spiritual properties, frankincense oil supports emotional balance, enhances meditation practices, and promotes healthy skin.

Essential Oil Storage and Shelf Life

Proper storage ensures the longevity and efficacy of essential oils:

1. Dark Glass Bottles: Store essential oils in dark-colored glass bottles to protect them from light and UV rays, which can degrade their quality over time.

2. Cool, Dark Place: Store oils in a cool, dark location away from direct sunlight and heat sources to prevent oxidation and maintain their potency.

3. Tight Seals: Ensure bottles are tightly sealed to prevent air exposure, which can accelerate oil oxidation and reduce shelf life.

4. Shelf Life: Most essential oils have a shelf life of 1-3 years when stored properly. Citrus oils like lemon or orange have shorter shelf lives, typically around 6-12 months.

Tools and Accessories for Essential Oil Use

Enhance your essential oil experience with the right tools and accessories:

1. Diffusers: Diffusers disperse essential oils into the air, promoting aromatherapy benefits throughout your home or workspace.

2. Roller Bottles: These are convenient for applying diluted essential oils directly to the skin, making them ideal for topical use.

3. Carrier Oils: Essential for diluting oils before topical application, carrier oils like jojoba, sweet almond, or fractionated coconut oil ensure safe and effective use.

4. Storage Boxes or Cases: Organize and protect your essential oil collection with storage boxes or cases designed to hold multiple bottles securely.

Continuing Education and Certification

Expand your knowledge and skills through ongoing education and certification:

1. Workshops and Courses: Attend workshops, seminars, or online courses offered by reputable organizations to deepen your understanding of essential oils, their properties, and applications.

2. Certification Programs: Consider pursuing certification as an aromatherapist or essential oil specialist through accredited programs that provide comprehensive training and certification.

3. Professional Associations: Join professional associations for aromatherapists and essential oil enthusiasts to access resources, networking opportunities, and continuing education.

Resources and Communities for Essential Oil Enthusiasts

Connect with like-minded individuals and access valuable resources:

1. Books and Publications: Here's a list of books that cover various aspects of essential oils, from their therapeutic uses to blending techniques and practical applications:

1. **"The Complete Book of Essential Oils and Aromatherapy" by Valerie Ann Worwood**

o A comprehensive guide covering essential oils, their properties, uses for health and well-being, and recipes for blends.

2. **"Essential Oil Safety: A Guide for Health Care Professionals" by Robert Tisserand and Rodney Young**

o An authoritative reference book on the safe use of essential oils, including safety guidelines, toxicity profiles, and recommended dilutions.

3. **"The Essential Life" by Total Wellness Publishing**

o A practical guidebook with detailed information on essential oils, their benefits, and various applications for health, beauty, and home care.

4. **"The Healing Power of Essential Oils" by Eric Zielinski, D.C.**

o Focuses on using essential oils for specific health conditions, including recipes for blends and practical tips for everyday use.

5. **"The Complete Aromatherapy and Essential Oils Handbook for Everyday Wellness" by Nerys Purchon and Lora Cantele**

o Offers a comprehensive overview of aromatherapy, essential oils, and therapeutic uses, with practical advice and recipes.

6. **"Essential Oils: Ancient Medicine" by Dr. Josh Axe, Jordan Rubin, and Ty Bollinger**

o Explores the historical uses of essential oils, their modern applications for health and wellness, and practical tips for incorporating oils into daily life.

7. **"The Aromatherapy Bible: The Definitive Guide to Using Essential Oils" by Gill Farrer-Halls**

o A detailed reference book covering essential oils, their properties, therapeutic uses, and guidance on blending oils for different purposes.

8. **"Aromatherapy for Healing the Spirit: Restoring Emotional and Mental Balance with Essential Oils" by Gabriel Mojay**

o Focuses on the psychological and emotional benefits of essential oils, including recipes for blends aimed at restoring emotional balance.

9. **"The Fragrant Mind: Aromatherapy for Personality, Mind, Mood, and Emotion" by Valerie Ann Worwood**

o Explores the psychological effects of essential oils and offers insights into using aromatherapy to support mental and emotional well-being.

10. **"The Essential Oil Maker's Handbook" by Bettina Malle and Helge Schmickl**

o A guide for those interested in making their own essential oils, including extraction methods, equipment needed, and practical advice.

These books provide valuable insights into the world of essential oils, from their therapeutic properties to practical applications and safety considerations. Whether you're a beginner or looking to deepen your knowledge, these resources offer a wealth of information to support your journey with essential oils.

2. Online Forums and Communities: Here's a list of online forums and communities where you can engage with others interested in essential oils, share experiences, ask questions, and learn more about aromatherapy:

1. **Essential Oil University Forum**

o A community-driven forum dedicated to essential oils, where users can discuss topics related to aromatherapy, safety, blending techniques, and more.

o Website: Essential Oil University Forum

2. **Aromatherapy and Essential Oils Forum on Reddit**

o A subreddit focused on aromatherapy and essential oils, featuring discussions on usage tips, DIY recipes, product recommendations, and scientific research.

o Website: Reddit - Aromatherapy and Essential Oils

3. **Aromaweb Aromatherapy and Essential Oils Community**

o A forum hosted by Aromaweb, offering discussions on essential oils, aromatherapy practices, blending recipes, and holistic health topics.

o Website: Aromaweb Forum

4. The Essential Oil Community Forum

o A platform where members can share knowledge, experiences, and resources related to essential oils, including safety guidelines, therapeutic uses, and product reviews.

o Website: The Essential Oil Community Forum

5. Facebook Groups

o There are numerous Facebook groups dedicated to essential oils, ranging from general discussions to specialized topics such as essential oils for specific health conditions or DIY recipes.

o Example: Essential Oil Enthusiasts Group

6. Natural Health Community Forums

o Various forums and communities focused on natural health and wellness often include sections dedicated to aromatherapy and essential oils.

o Example: Natural Health Forums

7. **Young Living and doTERRA Independent Distributor Communities**

o Independent distributors of Young Living and doTERRA often host forums and discussion boards where members can connect, share insights, and learn about essential oil products and usage.

These forums provide a platform for enthusiasts, practitioners, and beginners alike to learn, share experiences, and stay informed about the latest developments in the world of essential oils and aromatherapy.

3. Local Workshops and Meetups: Attend local meetups, workshops, or events hosted by aromatherapy enthusiasts or practitioners in your area to expand your knowledge and network.

Building your essential oil toolkit involves thoughtful selection of oils, proper storage practices, acquiring essential tools and accessories, pursuing education and certification opportunities, and connecting with supportive communities. By investing in your toolkit, you empower yourself to explore the benefits of aromatherapy, enhance well-being, and cultivate a deeper appreciation for the natural healing powers of essential oils. Whether you're a beginner or seasoned enthusiast, building a comprehensive toolkit sets the foundation for a fulfilling and enriching journey with essential oils.

Conclusion

In our exploration of essential oils, you've embarked on a journey of discovery—a journey that extends beyond mere practical applications into the realm of holistic wellness and self-care. You've learned to harness the natural healing properties of botanical essences, whether it's through creating customized blends for relaxation, enhancing skincare routines, or promoting a serene environment through diffusing oils.

Reflect on the moments when essential oils made a tangible difference in your life. Perhaps it was the calming influence of lavender during a stressful day, the soothing relief of peppermint for a tension headache, or the rejuvenating effects of citrus oils in your morning routine. These experiences not only illustrate the versatility of essential oils but also underscore their ability to nurture and restore balance.

Consider the personal growth that has unfolded along this journey. From learning about the chemistry of oils to understanding their emotional impacts, each insight has deepened your appreciation for nature's aromatic gifts. Embrace these insights as pillars of wisdom that enrich your holistic approach to health and wellness.

Future Trends and Innovations

Looking ahead, the future of essential oils is ripe with innovation and opportunity. As awareness of natural health alternatives grows, so does the demand for sustainable practices and ethical sourcing within the industry. Innovations in extraction methods, such as CO_2 extraction and steam distillation, continue to refine the purity and potency of oils, ensuring they retain their therapeutic benefits.

Emerging trends highlight the integration of aromatherapy into mainstream healthcare practices and wellness routines. From clinical settings to spa therapies and home environments, essential oils are increasingly recognized for their role in promoting relaxation, supporting immune function, and enhancing overall quality of life. Stay informed about these developments to make informed choices that align with your values and health goals.

Encouraging a Holistic Approach

Integrating essential oils into a balanced lifestyle goes beyond mere applications—it's about fostering a holistic approach to well-being. Embrace the synergy between aromatherapy and complementary practices such as mindfulness, nutrition, and physical activity. Create daily rituals that nourish the body, mind, and spirit, incorporating oils to enhance relaxation, focus, and vitality.

Consider the profound impact of aromatherapy on emotional wellness. Whether you're diffusing oils to create a calming atmosphere at home, incorporating them into meditation practices for inner peace, or using them in self-care routines for holistic rejuvenation, recognize the power of scent in nurturing emotional balance and resilience.

Embrace essential oils as natural allies in your journey towards wellness, empowering yourself to cultivate a lifestyle that prioritizes self-care and holistic health practices. By integrating oils into your daily routines with intention and mindfulness, you create a sanctuary of wellness that supports your overall well-being.

Final Thoughts and Inspirations

As we conclude this exploration of essential oils, let's celebrate the beauty and wisdom found in nature's aromatic treasures. Each drop of essential oil represents a gift from the earth, offering healing, rejuvenation, and a pathway to inner harmony. Embrace the journey with gratitude for the transformative power of aromatherapy in enriching our lives.

Reflect on the timeless wisdom embedded in botanical essences and their ability to nurture mind-body harmony. Whether you're exploring new blends, learning about aromatic traditions, or simply inhaling the fragrance of your favorite oils, cherish these moments as reminders of your connection to nature and the inherent healing potential it offers.

Inhale deeply, exhale gratitude, and carry forward the wisdom gained from your journey with essential oils. May your path be illuminated by the aromatic wonders of lavender fields, the invigorating zest of citrus groves, and the grounding presence of earthy oils, guiding you towards a life infused with vitality and serenity.

With heartfelt appreciation for the journey shared and inspiration for the road ahead, continue to explore, cherish, and celebrate the transformative essence of essential oils in every aspect of your life.

Appendix

Glossary of Terms Related to Essential Oils

As a comprehensive reference for readers exploring essential oils, this glossary provides detailed definitions and explanations of key terms commonly used in aromatherapy and essential oil practices.

Absorption: The process by which essential oils penetrate the skin or mucous membranes and enter the bloodstream to exert their therapeutic effects. Absorption rates vary based on the molecular size and lipid solubility of the essential oil.

Adulteration: The unethical practice of diluting or altering essential oils with synthetic chemicals or lower-quality oils to reduce costs, compromising their purity and therapeutic value. Adulterated oils may lack the beneficial properties of pure, unadulterated oils.

Analgesic: Essential oils with pain-relieving properties, effective for reducing discomfort from headaches, muscle aches, and minor injuries when applied topically or used in massage.

Anti-inflammatory: Essential oils that reduce inflammation and swelling when applied topically or inhaled. These oils are beneficial for conditions such as arthritis, muscle soreness, and skin irritation.

Anti-spasmodic: Essential oils that relax muscle spasms and cramps, providing relief from conditions such as menstrual cramps, digestive spasms, and muscular tension.

Antimicrobial: Essential oils with properties that inhibit the growth of microorganisms, including bacteria, viruses, and fungi. Antimicrobial oils are used in disinfectants, cleaning products, and for immune support.

Aromatic Profile: The unique scent characteristics and chemical composition of an essential oil, determined by its specific botanical source, growing conditions, and extraction method. Each essential oil has a distinct aromatic profile.

Aromatherapy: The therapeutic use of aromatic plant extracts (essential oils) to promote physical, emotional, and psychological well-being. Aromatherapy techniques include inhalation, topical application, and diffusion.

Blending: The art and science of combining multiple essential oils and carrier oils to create customized blends tailored to specific therapeutic or aromatic purposes. Blending involves understanding the properties and interactions of different oils for desired effects.

Carrier Oil: A neutral, base oil used to dilute essential oils before topical application to reduce the risk of irritation and enhance absorption. Common carrier oils include jojoba oil, coconut oil, and almond oil.

CO2 Extraction: An advanced extraction method that uses carbon dioxide under high pressure to isolate essential oils from plant material. CO2 extraction preserves the full spectrum of volatile compounds, resulting in oils of high purity and potency.

Cold Pressing: A method of extracting essential oils from citrus fruits by mechanically pressing the fruit rinds to release aromatic oils. This method is used for oils like lemon, orange, and grapefruit essential oils.

Dilution Ratio: The proportion of essential oil to carrier oil used in blends, expressed as a ratio (e.g., 2% dilution means 2 drops of essential oil per 98 drops of carrier oil). Dilution ratios ensure safe and effective use of essential oils on the skin.

Digestive: Essential oils that support healthy digestion and relieve digestive discomfort, used topically on the abdomen or inhaled to promote gastrointestinal health.

Diffusion: The process of dispersing essential oils into the air for inhalation, typically using devices such as ultrasonic diffusers, nebulizers, or aromatherapy candles. Diffusion allows for the therapeutic inhalation of essential oil vapors.

Emulsifier: A substance that helps mix essential oils with water-based products, facilitating the creation of aromatherapy sprays, lotions, or bath products. Emulsifiers ensure even distribution of oils in water-based formulas.

EOBBD (Essential Oil Botanical and Biochemical Diversity): A quality standard ensuring essential oils are sourced from specific botanical species and exhibit biochemical properties characteristic of the species. EOBBD-certified oils guarantee authenticity and therapeutic efficacy.

Expectorant: Essential oils that promote the expulsion of mucus from the respiratory tract, aiding in clearing congestion and supporting respiratory health.

GC-MS Analysis: Gas Chromatography-Mass Spectrometry analysis, a scientific method used to analyze and verify the chemical composition of essential oils. GC-MS analysis identifies individual components and confirms the authenticity and purity of oils.

Hydrosol: Also known as floral waters or plant waters, hydrosols are by-products of the steam distillation process of essential oils. They contain diluted water-soluble aromatic compounds and are used in skincare, aromatherapy, and as natural spritzers.

Mucolytic: Essential oils that help break down mucus and clear congestion in the respiratory system, beneficial for respiratory conditions such as colds, coughs, and sinusitis.

Neat Application: Applying undiluted essential oils directly to the skin, which is generally not recommended except in specific circumstances or with certain oils known for their safety in neat use, such as lavender or tea tree oil.

Organic: Essential oils derived from plants grown without synthetic pesticides, fertilizers, or genetic modifications, certified by organic standards organizations. Organic oils promote sustainable farming practices and minimize exposure to harmful chemicals.

Patch Test: A method to test skin sensitivity to essential oils by applying a diluted oil to a small area of skin and monitoring for any adverse reactions before broader use.

Patch testing helps determine individual sensitivity and potential allergic reactions.

Phototoxicity: A skin reaction caused by exposure to certain essential oils (particularly citrus oils) followed by exposure to sunlight or UV light. Phototoxic oils can cause increased skin sensitivity, burns, or pigmentation changes if not used with caution.

Steam Distillation: A traditional method of extracting essential oils from plant material using steam to release and collect aromatic compounds. Steam distillation is used for oils derived from flowers, leaves, and other plant parts.

Stimulant: Essential oils that increase alertness, mental clarity, and physical energy when inhaled or applied topically. Stimulant oils are used to combat fatigue and enhance cognitive function.

Synergy: The combined effect of essential oils working together harmoniously to produce a greater therapeutic benefit than the sum of their individual effects. Synergy is often achieved through blending complementary oils for specific therapeutic purposes.

Therapeutic Grade: A term sometimes used by essential oil companies to imply a high quality and purity level suitable for therapeutic use, though it lacks standardized regulation. Look for oils that are tested for purity and meet specific quality standards.

Tonifying: Essential oils that strengthen and invigorate bodily tissues and systems, promoting overall health and vitality when used regularly.

This glossary serves as a valuable resource for understanding essential oil terminology, enhancing reader knowledge, and promoting safe and informed usage in aromatherapy practices.

Did You Enjoy This Book?

Dear Reader,

I hope this message finds you well. I wanted to take a moment to express my sincere gratitude for choosing to read Essential Oils Unveiled: A Comprehensive Guide to Natural Healing and Wellness. It means the world to me that you've invested your time and trust in my work.

If you found Essential Oils Unveiled: A Comprehensive Guide to Natural Healing and Wellness enjoyable and valuable, I would be immensely grateful if you could spare a few moments to leave a review on Amazon, Goodreads, etc. Your feedback not only helps other readers discover the book but also provides valuable insights for me as an author.

Whether it's a brief comment about what you liked most, how the book impacted you, or simply your overall impression, your review would make a significant difference. Your honest opinion is invaluable in helping me grow as a writer and in reaching more readers.

Thank you so much for your support and for being a part of this journey with me. Your reviews truly mean the world to me.

Sarah Burkhartt

Warmest regards,

Sarah Burkhartt

Three Isles Publishing

About the Author

Sarah Burkhartt is a passionate advocate for natural healing and wellness, with a deep expertise in aromatherapy and essential oils. As a certified aromatherapist and holistic health practitioner, Sarah has dedicated her career to exploring the therapeutic benefits of plant-based remedies, particularly through the use of essential oils. Her journey into the world of aromatherapy began over two decades ago, driven by a desire to promote holistic approaches to health.

Sarah is known for her comprehensive understanding of essential oil profiles, blending techniques, and their applications for various health conditions. Her approach emphasizes the importance of sustainable practices and quality standards in sourcing and using essential oils.

In addition to her practice as an aromatherapist, Sarah is a prolific writer and educator in the field of natural health. Her commitment to empowering individuals to integrate essential oils into their daily lives for improved well-being is reflected in her accessible yet authoritative writing style.

"Essential Oils Unveiled: A Comprehensive Guide to Natural Healing and Wellness" is Sarah Burkhartt's latest endeavor to share her wealth of knowledge and practical insights with readers seeking to harness the power of nature for health and vitality. Through this book, Sarah aims to inspire and educate, guiding readers on a transformative journey towards holistic wellness through the therapeutic use of essential oils.

Sarah resides in a serene countryside setting, where she continues to explore new applications and advancements in aromatherapy while nurturing her passion for sustainable living and natural health practices.